THE NATURAL PHARMACY PRODUCT GUIDE

RICHARD ISRAEL

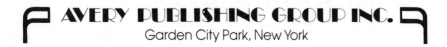
AVERY PUBLISHING GROUP INC.

Garden City Park, New York

The health procedures and opinions in this book are based on the training, personal experiences, and research of the author. Because each person and situation is unique, the editor and the publisher urge the reader to check with a qualified health professional before using any procedure where there is any question as to its appropriateness.

The publisher does not advocate the use of any particular diet, but believes the information presented in this book should be available to the public.

Because there is always some risk involved, the author and publisher are not responsible for any adverse effects or consequences resulting from the use of any of the suggestions, preparations, or procedures in this book. Please do not use the book if you are unwilling to assume the risk. Feel free to consult a physician or other qualified health professional. It is a sign of wisdom, not cowardice, to seek a second or third opinion.

Cover Design: Rudy Shur and Martin Hochberg
Original Text Artwork: Michael Apici
In-House Editors: Carolyn Sofia, Marie Caratozzolo
Typesetters: Straight Creek Company, Denver, CO

Library of Congress Cataloging-in-Publication Data

Israel, Richard,
     The natural pharmacy product guide / Richard Israel,
       p. cm.
     Includes bibliographical references and index.
     ISBN 0-89529-465-6
     1. Homeopathy—Materia medica and therapeutics.   2. Holistic
     medicine.   I. Title.
     RX601.I84   1991
     615.5'32—dc20   90-24377
                                                                  CIP

Printed in the United States of America

10   9   8   7   6   5   4   3   2   1

Contents

PART TWO: HEALING PARTNERS—NATURAL MEDICINES

Acknowledgements

My thanks to all those people who care enough about the quality of life to demand good products for consumption and healing. For it is the desire of caring people that brought about the creation of the many fine natural products available on the shelves today. It was that same need that drove me to learn and record what you will find in this book, and it is with great pleasure that I am able to share this information and the knowledge of these wonderful tools with all of you.

And also my thanks to Dwight Howard, Jeanie Zazzi, Everett McGuire, and the manufacturers of the fine products listed in this book for their valuable help.

And most of all, my love and thanks to Eileen, whose patience and support allowed me the time and space to create this work.

—R.I.

Foreword

Having been involved with and interested in natural health care for many years, I am now glad to be able to add this book to my library. Often, we are afraid to question our medical institutions when dealing with the everyday occurrences of minor sore throats, headaches, scrapes, and other common problems. I feel we should be more aware of the safer, gentler choices available to us.

As we go to the drug store to pick up a sore throat lozenge, do we know about the possible side effects of the ingredients on the label? If we could choose a safe alternative that would give us relief without endangering our health, which would be the most sensible choice? I would want the safer product when the condition is not serious enough to require a doctor's advice. And if I need to consult a physician, I want to be aware enough to ask my doctor if a safer product might be as effective.

For those of us who are interested in increasing our awareness to take better care of our health and the health of our loved ones, this text is a timely tool. Presented in a down-to-earth format, it not only teaches about the useful products available, but also illuminates the magnificence of the human body and its self-healing potential. This book has provided a convenient guide to effective nutritional aids that can be employed for the everyday ailments that confront us. I look forward to many years of enjoyment and use from this practical reference.

Everett McGuire
President, Stress Management Systems
Healing Massage Instructor
Professional Sports Massage Therapist

Preface

When I decided to write this volume, my wishes were to provide a tool for both those people familiar with natural healing products and those who have relatively little knowledge of the subject. I found myself faced with the dilemma of creating a book that was easy and enjoyable for the novice to read and understand, and yet was, at the same time, documented with adequate scientific data.

My intentions were to write in an informal manner so as not to bore or confuse the individuals just beginning to investigate the realm of more wholesome healing alternatives. At the same time, I have tried to support this information with some substance, as I wouldn't want anyone to accept my opinions without verifying the facts.

I've selected the products I have found to be superior in their categories from my many years of experience with the health industry. I've also tried not to be biased except in my own experience with these products. In my opinion, a reference book of this kind is needed to help transform the concepts about quality of first-aid treatment in the home to a safer, healthier level. This text concerns those conditions for which we tend to treat ourselves and our family members by simply buying non-prescription products at the local drug store. We all deserve to know what exists in the way of safe and effective alternatives to the preparations offered by the chemical pharmaceutical companies.

Many of us have been intimidated by the medical profession and the pharmaceutical companies in a way that often induces fear when we consider trying alternatives to these established institutions. These professionals offer a great deal of help in many serious situations and I don't mean to say we don't need their valuable contributions. Again, the alternatives I want to introduce you to are for minor ailments where a doctor's advice is not usually required. For these occurrences, a little education can enable your common sense to direct you. As George Sheehan, M.D., a well-known cardiologist, once said,

> There is no reason why a profession that learned from a soldier how to treat gout, from a sailor how to keep off scurvy, from a milkmaid how to prevent smallpox, should now require that an individual have an M.D. after his name before it will listen to what he has to say on the subject of medicine.[1]

I attempted to include for you the information I would want if I were to relearn this subject. I also tried to provide this material in a comfortable and practical format. I hope you will find this book to be an interesting and informative adventure as well as a valuable tool for selecting products for your health and the health of your loved ones.

—R.I.
Boulder, Colorado

Introduction

With the many changes that have come along as we approach the end of the twentieth century, an awareness of the quality of our environment has become much more widespread. Announcers on radio stations in many of our major cities might say, "This is a high-pollution day. If you have a respiratory problem, you should stay inside until the air quality is at a safer level." Our TV news coverage informs us of agricultural areas where the rampant use of chemical fertilizers and pesticides has made much of our ground water unfit to drink. We learn that many areas of our oceans are also suffering from pollution. Off the shores of highly populated coastal areas, the quality of the surviving sea life as a food product is questionable.

It is also difficult to have a great deal of confidence in food products with long, ominous, unfamiliar names on their ingredient labels. How do we know what we are ingesting when we eat something containing polysorbate 60, ethylenediamine tetraacetate, or glucono-delta-a-lactone? We find that many products proclaimed safe by our government agencies eventually turn out to have unexpected and tragic side effects. All the input from this time of increased media coverage has made Americans increasingly conscious of the food they eat.

As people become aware of the effects on their bodies of overly processed and chemically laden foods, they become more conscious consumers. They are investigating naturally grown and minimally processed foods, reading labels more carefully, and questioning the quality of the foods they select for themselves and their families more thoroughly.

As awareness grows among consumers, the industries that serve these consumers respond and grow as well. As a participant and observer, I have watched the natural foods industry develop over the past twenty years. I have also watched the people involved grow in their knowledge as more information and research has become available. I found the health food store (mainly a pill shop) of the 1950s confronted by the wide selection of grocery products found in the natural foods store of the 1960s. These early natural food markets were often run by unprofessional types with only their limited knowledge of better food alternatives and a sincere desire to improve availability of quality foods for themselves and others as their motivation. Unfortunately, these early stores were often unorganized, sometimes not too clean, and very limited in their selection of products.

The natural foods industry has grown in leaps and bounds since that time. Today's stores are full of products that have become more and more sophisticated. Fifteen years ago, of the few natural food products available, many really were not very tasty and at best, boring. Creative manufacturers have learned to duplicate many of our favorite foods with surprisingly good replication of texture and taste, while improving the quality of the ingredients. Even the packaging has changed from a bland or "funky" motif, to some of the beautiful graphic designs we find on the shelves today. As information continues to come to the surface, better ingredients are used in these products. Many of the big supermarket chains now have health food sections and they watch the natural food markets for new, fast-moving items to add to their shelves.

As consumers become more aware of the foods they put in their bodies, they also seek better medicinal products. We hear a lot about the potential side effects of many chemical pharmaceutical medicines. Many lose the faith they once had in the medical profession and its prescriptions. As a result, these individuals become increasingly concerned and begin to search for more natural alternatives to standard medicinal products. At the same time the natural grocery industry has become more sophisticated, so has the natural healing category of this industry. Natural healing products, as tools for relief of minor ailments, have grown in both number of products and effectiveness in recent years.

I'm not proclaiming that conventional medical doctors and their prescription drugs have no place in health care. The purpose of this book is not to prescribe products to cure ailments, as I am not a medical doctor and am obviously not authorized to do such a thing. By all means I encourage any reader to consult a physician if he or she is experiencing any prolonged or serious disorder or is presently taking some prescription formula. It is my opinion that people should not toss out their medications and start with only natural products, but should educate themselves in natural health care first. They can then experiment with nutritional alternatives in cooperation with their doctors to see if their body defenses strengthen to a point where less of their prescribed medicines are needed.

The sole purpose of this book is to inform you of some fine alternative products that exist for everyday minor disturbances. In most cases, you probably wouldn't consult a physician to treat conditions that fall into this category. The products in this book are considered nutritional substances or over-the-counter (OTC) drugs. An OTC drug is a non-toxic substance taken for an ailment that does not require a doctor's diagnosis or monitoring and that will resolve itself eventually without medical intervention. At no time do I mean to indicate that these products will cure an illness or injury, but rather that these products are nutritional supplements capable of making the body stronger and more able to ward off unhealthy conditions.

I put this writing together to make you aware of a few products that you can purchase without a prescription, just as you are able to purchase aspirins or laxatives. The difference is that the ingredients in these medicinals tend to be beneficial for your body as a whole. Most of these products are completely safe. Be sure to read the labels carefully for any warnings or dosage instructions.

At one time, individuals wanting a more natural product to treat an ailment would refer to a book on herbs for a remedy. Then they would go to an herb shop or a natural foods store and purchase the appropriate dried herb. Perhaps they would then take a quantity of the herb and make a tea to drink or prepare it in some other way.

Unfortunately, consumers had no way of knowing much about the herb they purchased. Not only might they have questions about the dosage to use, but also about the herb's quality or the amount of the active ingredients in it. Two herb plants of the same species growing only feet apart may be very different in composition. At times consumers may not even get the herb they thought they were purchasing because many herbs look alike and the person harvesting the herb may have mistaken the identity of the plant.

Another factor that can affect herbs is the processing and storage conditions. If the herbs were subjected to extreme conditions (heat, sunlight, etc.), the quality of the finished product can be affected. So suppose you have studied your herb books and have your preparation work perfected. How do you know how much of the active ingredients, the substances that will help the condition you are treating, are actually in your preparation?

Well, luckily there is a solution to this problem. Nowadays there are reputable herb companies, some of which are registered as pharmaceutical companies, under the sharp eye of the FDA. These companies must meet stringent requirements with every item that leaves their manufacturing facilities. In Europe, Japan, China, and elsewhere, herbs and other natural remedies have been accepted medicines for decades and significant research documentation indicating their effectiveness is readily available. In recent years, many of these preparations have become available in this country.

So now there are healing products out there with natural ingredients from reputable companies. How do consumers choose which of these products are good for them? That's where I hope this manual will help. Over the past two decades, while being involved in the health product and healing industries, I have become aware of some exceptional tools for everyday problems and ailments. It is this information that I want to share with you.

Again, I'm not saying that the products listed in this book will heal your particular condition, as what works for one may not be the perfect tool for another. Any particular symptom can be caused by a number of different conditions or imbalances. For example, a sinus condition could be a result of an allergy, an infection, or the elimination of toxic substances by the body. Because of the complexity of each of our individual make-ups, we can't expect that all these products will perform well for each and every one of us at any given time. Even standard medicine does not have this sort of a track record. At least this text can give you a place to start in choosing from the wide selection of products available to the consumer today.

I am not professing that the products listed in this book are the only beneficial products available. To list all the superb products on the shelves would make this volume too lengthy and cumbersome and I want it to be an easy-to-use, helpful tool. I simply feel that some of the products I'm familiar with are exceptional enough that I wouldn't hesitate to share my knowledge of them with my friends. My hope is, that when you are finished reading this book, you will not only be one of my friends, but will also be able to successfully stock your own home medicine cabinet with safe, effective natural products.

Part One

Health and Natural Healing: The Basics

In this section I will introduce you to natural healing methods and ideologies as well as some basic guidelines regarding the capabilities of certain foods to contribute to your health, either in a beneficial or detrimental way. You will also be familiarized with the types of products I will be addressing specifically later in the book. My hope is that you will gain an understanding of the natural healing processes and the type of foods and products that support and stimulate these processes in the body. Armed with this information, the decision how to structure your diet will be in your hands.

1

Fundamentals of Natural Healing

The human body is a very unique and special instrument designed to allow an individual to move around in this world and to experience many amazing and beautiful things. To smell a rose, to feel the warmth of the sun, or see the radiance of a perfect sunset are all abilities we generally take for granted. However, if we take the time to experience such things and also allow time to ponder how special it is that we can accomplish these actions, we begin to glimpse how fantastic this human life really is. But at the same time the body allows us to do all this and more, it has an unbelievable ability to keep its own mechanism running quite smoothly and, in most cases, to correct the injustices inflicted upon it by both the environment and our poor eating habits. With its elaborate system of natural defenses, the human body is quite an impressive instrument!

If we eat something that is toxic, mechanisms in our bodies react to try to remove the substance in many different ways. If what we have ingested is extremely toxic, we might find our bodies responding with diarrhea or even vomiting. In many cases, we may find our internal systems heating up with fevers in order to oxidize the toxins and push them from the body with flows of perspiration. This increase in body temperature also speeds the blood flow, allowing healing systems to move quickly to a distressed area and encouraging the dangerous toxins to be eliminated as rapidly as possible. Other systems may initiate such responses as coughing, gagging, sneezing, and many kinds of mucus secretions, depending on the nature of the toxic accumulations.

With minute quantities of toxic material that can't be removed easily from the body, the substances will often accumulate in the feet or hands. This mechanism keeps the dangerous substances as far away from the vital organs as possible. This is why you may feel sharp pains when someone massaging your feet presses firmly on certain areas on the sole of your foot. These tender areas can represent toxic accumulations. A good massage therapist knows that if he or she does too much work on someone's feet, excess toxins may be released and the individual could have a "healing reaction" that may appear as cold symptoms or some other release of the body's detrimental accumulations.

In the case of biological invasions, such as a virus or a bacterial infection, the circulatory system carries antibodies and engulfing white blood cells to attack the invaders. The liver acts as a highly discriminating filter pulling many toxins out of the blood stream and, in some cases, neutralizing them. In cases where the liver cannot neutralize these substances, they can accumulate and cause damage to this important organ. The spleen is well known for its function as a contributor to the body's immune system. It produces antibodies, increases the number of neutrophils (a type of white blood cell with the ability to engulf harmful bacteria), and filters foreign matter out of the blood. Such matter may include bacteria and parasites killed by white blood cells and blood cells that have become old or damaged.[1]

Some organs or groups of organs act to keep elements in the body at safe and optimum levels. For example, salt, sugar, and various hormones must maintain a delicate balance in the body. These organs, aided by many feedback stimuli, maintain certain levels of many tissue nutrients to protect the body and allow it to function properly.

As you can see, the human body is a complex organization of protection systems dedicated to preserving the health of the entire organism. It only makes sense that with all these sophisticated battling systems as our allies, maybe our best defense is to keep these systems working at their optimum capacity. Hippocrates, an ancient Greek physician known as "The Father of Medicine," once said, "A disease is to be cured naturally by man's own power, and physicians help it."

What do these systems need in order to operate at their best? Another great man of medicine, Shin-huang-ti, who compiled the fundamentals of Chinese medicine in the Ch'in era of China, said, "It is diet which maintains true health and becomes the best drug." What we require is just the regular good old stuff we all know about. Good food, exercise, a good mental attitude, and sometimes a little extra attention to keep this living wonder we inhabit working properly. This extra attention may be a vitamin, herb, or food supplement that we are lacking; a little bodywork; removal from a stressful situation; the care of a qualified doctor or therapist; or some other regime. The important thing is to be in touch with our bodies enough to recognize when some extra help is needed. When Mr. Franklin said, "An ounce of prevention is worth a pound of cure," he was being not only profound, but practical as well.

The common cold is such a routine occurrence that almost everyone is affected by it at least once a year. According to Robert S. Mendelsohn, M. D., the many theories surrounding it are often grouped into two categories: the moral category and the viral category. According to the moral theory, you caught a cold because you didn't take care of yourself. For example, mothers insist their children caught colds because they didn't wear coats or mittens. According to the viral theory, those children would have caught colds whether they had worn mittens or not, just because the "bug" was going around. Obviously, there is some truth to both theories, but what about children who didn't wear mittens when the virus was rampant and still didn't catch colds?

Some people have what is called a strong constitution while other people have what is called a weak constitution. Those with strong constitutions seem to ward off illness better than their more delicate counterparts. The strength of our constitutions can be traced to genetic factors, just as dark hair and light hair can. Unfortunately, if we have weak constitutions, we have no control over them. But our genes are by no means the only factors that contribute to our susceptibility to illness and disease.

Our environment, habits, and diet also contribute considerably to our state of health. Many of us find that, as we become older, we no longer have the immunity from ailments we had in our youth. Often, we find that we can no longer eat all the things we once never had to think about twice. We may find ourselves on restrictive diets. Sensitivities to sugar or salt and allergies to wheat, corn, and dairy products become more and more common. Years of mistreating our bodies have finally taken their toll.

The earlier we respect the gift of a human body and educate ourselves in the proper care of this complex mechanism, the better off we will be in the later years of our lives. It always astounds me to consider what our bodies can put up with. Isn't it truly amazing, how much abuse most human bodies can endure before completely breaking down?

Just living in this world in this day and age, we subject our bodies to many of the influences of a polluted environment. The air in most parts of our continent is not particulary clean and the foods we eat, even if we are selective, usually contain tiny amounts of toxic substances. These substances may be pesticides or chemical fertilizers on agricultural crops or the numerous products made from these crops. Even unsprayed crops may pick up harmful chemicals from the contaminated ground water in our agricultural areas. We may be ingesting steroids or other unnatural compounds that are fed to our livestock on a daily basis. Many of our oceans are becoming polluted as the unclean waters of our rivers carry our waste to the sea, making many of our sea foods heavily laden with undesirable contaminates. Many of our highly processed foods are filled with questionable chemicals in order to increase their shelf lives, change their color, or just to keep ingredients from separating. Many of these unnatural substances may accumulate in the body tissues and cause problems when they become too concentrated.

The stress of our fast pace of living also has a detrimental effect on the ability of our bodily defenses to work at their best. Working under fluorescent lighting, which does not contain the full spectrum of light, is said to deplete our bodies of Vitamin A, an element that aids the blood's ability to supply oxygen to the cells. Stress is known to use up the B-Complex vitamins at a very rapid rate, leaving our nervous systems feeling "on edge." Again, there are many factors affecting our health that we have no control over. But if there are a few things we can do to keep the damage at a minimum, isn't it worth our while to consider these options?

Just to set the record straight, I'm definitely not a purist when it comes to diet. I believe one can become a little too tight about diet and lose the fun of enjoying some of the delicious taste sensations out there. At the same time, I prefer to be a practical man rather than a complete fool when it comes to indulging myself. I usually go by the 95 percent rule. I believe that if I eat good, wholesome food, free of preservatives and additives most of the time, it won't hurt me to indulge in some purely decadent foods once in a while.

Now if you are ill, you may need to be on a strict diet for a while in order to bring yourself back to a healthy state. But in the case of maintenance, to keep your body healthy, I feel some folks become a little too fanatical about their diets and often make themselves ill simply because they are too rigid and lose their balance. Their fear of harmful foods results in stress, which may lead to illness. You don't need to add more stress to your life by trying to eat in too regimented a fashion.

Of course, you have to remain in touch with your own body and it's your decision just how much abuse you care to inflict on yourself. But keep in mind that if you overdo it, chances are you may have to suffer the consequences at some time in the future. Do you think twice about taking care of your automobile if you want it to run properly? You wouldn't fill your tank with dirty gasoline, because if you did, sooner or later something would get clogged up and the car would fail to run properly. The human machine is a delicately engineered instrument and needs similar attention and care. I don't intend to tell you how to eat or what to eat; but in Chapter 3, I will put down a few guidelines that you may find useful. I sincerely feel that health begins with educating ourselves about healthy foods and healthy attitudes.

In my opinion, this book describes many exceptional healing products, some of which, hopefully, will help many of you with common ailments. But let's give credit where credit is due. The real healing element is the human body with all of its intricate defense systems. The natural medicines merely act as supporting partners in this endeavor, providing the necessary nutrients and energies needed to allow these systems to perform optimally.

A Holistic Approach to Health

Medical practitioners often look at obvious symptoms such as headaches or congestion and work to suppress these symptoms. It is a common theory that if relief is provided for the symptom then the person is healed. Sometimes, when the same conditions arise again and again, even stronger drugs are given to subdue the discomfort. Many strong drugs have been developed because they relieve symptoms quickly. Unfortunately, in many cases these medicines merely decrease discomfort or make abnormal visual signs, such as skin rashes, swelling, etc., disappear while never really dealing with the cause of the disorder.

Pain, discomfort, and such abnormal visual signs are nature's methods of signaling us when there is a problem that needs our attention. Even though pain can be an unpleasant experience, without its warning signals we could be unaware of an injury or illness. Perhaps an illness could progress to an even more dangerous extreme without our having taken proper curative actions. In this way, the signs of a disorder, though we may view them as a scourge, are but another example of nature's means of protecting us from harm.

I firmly believe that discomfort should be relieved and that the ability to do so is a necessary attribute of a medicine. Unfortunately, if the deeper cause of a problem is not also dealt with, then, even though the symptom disappears, it may recur again and again. The products mentioned in this book have helped many people attain relief from the uncomfortable symptoms of various health problems. Because most of these medicines are also foods, they may relieve discomfort while they nourish the body systems so health might be restored. I hope that some of you readers can achieve benefits from the use of the products I will be introducing you to.

Health practitioners with a more naturalistic foundation tend to take a more holistic approach to healing. This means that they try to treat the symptoms of a disorder as well as the causes. While they look carefully at the physical body, they are also aware that other factors may contribute to poor health. Mental or emotional imbalances due to poor diet, allergies, lack of exercise, environmental factors, stressful living, or intense work situations may all lead to physical disorders. In other words, natural health practitioners make an effort to look at the whole picture when dealing with their patients.

"Holistic" derives from the word "whole." So when we talk about holistic medicine, we are talking about a consideration for the whole organism and an approach to bringing about a condition of total health, not just stopping a symptom. Symptomatic medicine, on the other hand, can sometimes be like putting a Band-Aid on a cancerous skin ulcer. If you can't see the problem anymore, then it no longer exists! Using a holistic approach, a doctor would suggest not only medicines but dietary supplements, a good exercise program (depending on the condition of the patient, of course), possibly some physical therapy or body work, and perhaps something to help the mental attitude such as affirmations, mental exercises, or even counseling.

Fortunately, the importance of good nutrition in health care is becoming more and more common knowledge in the medical community. In 1988, United States Surgeon General C. Everett Koop issued the most comprehensive study of diet and health ever undertaken by the U.S. government. This 712-page report, drawing on over 2,500 scientific articles, contained many recommendations that natural foods advocates had proclaimed for years. Among its recommendations: Americans should cut their intake of saturated fats, sugar, alcohol, and salt, while increasing exercise and consumption of complex carbohydrates and fiber. Koop went on to say, "Your choice of diet can influence your long-term health prospects more than any other action you might take."[2]

Burton Kalliman, Director of Science and Technology for the National Nutritional Foods Association (NNFA), comments, "The report repeats dietary advice which is basically identical to what the health food industry has given for many years and other organizations have lately adopted as the 'prudent diet.'"

Regardless of who said it first, it is comforting to know that some progress is being made in the education of health professionals as to the importance of proper nutrition. This breakthrough has brought more individuals into the health food markets who would have never entered them before. Who knows, maybe it will open the door for more professionals to consider a more holistic approach to health.

Drugs

The *Merriam-Webster Dictionary* defines "drug" as a "substance used as or in a medicine." Under this definition, medicinal foods such as herbs would be classified as drugs. But to distinguish between the chemicals synthesized in the laboratory and the more natural preparations that are used in the treatment of injuries and disease symptoms, I will refer to the former as "drugs" and the latter as "natural medicines."

The traditional American approach to medicine in this century is to "control" disease rather than aid the body's natural systems to combat health problems. It was not until very recently that the medical establishment began seriously to look at the body's own immune system. The medical community is now recognizing immune responses as a key in the defense against some serious diseases, including Acquired Immune Deficiency Syndrome (AIDS) and cancer. In the case of cardiovascular disease, the medical profession is beginning to recognize the role nutrition plays in preventing this problem. But, for the most part, standard medicine has tried to arrest or control the symptoms of disease rather than treat the body as a holistic unit with sophisticated systems for regulating health. Because of this orientation to health, doctors have been willing to prescribe many chemical compounds that have been in existence for no more than a decade or two. What are the long-range ramifications of this practice? Or, for that matter, what damage has already been done as a result of this practice?

According to Robert S. Mendelsohn, M.D., author of the book *How to Raise a Healthy Child . . . In Spite of Your Doctor*, it is rare that a doctor investigates the tests to which a drug or a treatment has been subjected before he uses it on his patients. In 1979, of the 30 most frequently prescribed drugs labeled ineffective by the Food and Drug Administration (FDA), more than half were prescribed for children. Dr. Mendelsohn claims that 90 percent of the drugs prescribed by pediatricians are unnecessary and costly risks to the child who takes them.[3]

In the case of diethylstilbestrol (DES, for short), it was used by over two million females to prevent miscarriages even though earlier research in the 1950s indicated it to be ineffective for this purpose.[4] In 1971, researchers announced that some of the female offspring of women who took DES were developing vaginal and cervical cancer at a rate thousands of times higher than the normal statistics. This drug was still being prescribed in the late 1980s as a morning-after contraceptive, another condition for which there seems to be little proof of its effectiveness.[5] This same drug is readily given to cattle, and millions of meat-eating Americans are ingesting it daily. In 1975, Massachusetts Senator Edward M. Kennedy tried to have DES banned, but the drug companies had his case set aside saying they did not have adequate time for a hearing.[6] After this attempt, no more was heard about taking it off the market. It seems a bit unusual that the FDA wastes little time investigating herbs, L-tryptophan, and other natural healing substances while it allows drugs like DES with proven health hazards to be freely administered by the medical profession.

The truth is that medical science in America is a very complex and unique system that combines politics and economics in a way that supports and promotes the products of the powerful pharmaceutical companies. It is not enough if a product achieves results, it must also be profitable. If the healing agent is a naturally occurring botanical, it cannot be patented and the drug company cannot control the rights to it. If they cannot control the rights to a product, they cannot make the profits they want and they won't bother to spend the millions of dollars it takes to develop and market the item.

Unfortunately, the problem doesn't stop there. Because profit is such an important concern to these corporations, they enlist strong lobbies to discredit natural products. One effective tactic has been to label the natural products as "unproven." Professionals interpret this to mean "not effective" or even "dangerous" even though countries other than ours may have plenty of documentation supporting the effectiveness of these substances. Unfortunately, when determining product safety, our government agencies do not recognize research data from competent researchers in other countries.

Our own regulatory agencies have, unfortunately, evolved into an entity that is so closely involved with the pharmaceutical companies that it is difficult to see who the government agency is really serving. Though they appear as agencies dedicated to protecting the nation's health, it is hard not to question some of the decisions they have made concerning many drugs.

The last ten years have shown a decrease in the number of mortalities from cardiovascular diseases. The drug companies boasted that new drugs developed for hypertension were responsible for fewer deaths. A recent study was done on men in the 35-to-57-year-old age bracket. All were generally healthy, but in a high-risk category because of high blood pressure, elevated cholesterol levels, or smoking habits. They were observed for ten years and, after a few additional years to correlate all the data, the results were reported. They were startling. The men with high blood pressure who received medication were dying *sooner* than the men who received no drugs. On top of that, it was found that the more drugs that were used by an individual, the higher his rate of death.[7]

In 1985 alone, approximately 1.5 billion prescriptions were written in the United States. That's 7.5 prescriptions for every person residing in this country. This adds up to approximately 600 pills per individual, including infants. According to Dr. Kurt W. Donsbach, one of America's foremost nutritionists and health educators, approximately 10 percent of the 30 million people admitted to hospitals are there because of adverse drug reactions. One large hospital attributed 25 percent of its in-house deaths to adverse drug reactions.[8]

Now I believe that there is definitely a place for modern synthetic medicine, and technology is definitely something that can contribute to our well-being, but shouldn't *all* the possibilities for treating a health problem be addressed? It seems sensible in less urgent situations to try safer, more natural approaches to healing before resorting to more drastic chemical approaches that increase the chances of developing harmful side effects.

2

Tools and Methods of Natural Healing

There are many schools of natural healing. Some healing methods, such as the use of herbs, have been developed and used since ancient times. Others, such as the science of homeopathy, have been in use for only two centuries, a relatively short time when you look at our history as human beings. As this world of separate nations becomes more of a world community, other methods of natural healing used for many decades or centuries by non-Western cultures are just recently becoming known to Western man. Acupuncture and certain bodywork techniques are examples.

Our modern technologies can also open new doors and can improve upon some of the traditional medicines. Modern scientific techniques can allow us to develop new methods of treating patients, and if done sensitively, need not compromise the basics of natural medicine. Increased availability of healing knowledge and increased supply have also led to the development of new and effective formulas and techniques to aid the natural healing practitioner. All of these factors make this a very exciting time to learn about the natural healing tools available to us.

The Use of Herbs as Healing Agents

Some people think the use of herbs as medicines is a new idea, perhaps begun by the back-to-the-land movement of the 1960s or a group of back-to-nature people. On the contrary, herbalism has been around for quite a long time. A few years back I was asked by a representative of the Colorado Department of Agriculture to address a group of farmers about marketing organic farming products. This group had been assembled to allow the troubled farming community to look at specialty crop alternatives and I was one of a panel of speakers. I began by saying "organic farming" was once known by another name. It was once called "farming"! It has only been in recent years, since the development of agricultural chemicals, that we've used methods other than natural means to feed crops and combat insect pests. The same is true of the use of chemical medicines. In the scope of history, this practice is really only a recent development.

Many of our early ancestors, using instinct, experience, taste, and observation, discovered many useful items among the selection found in the plant kingdom. So meticulous was their investigation that there is indication that most of the 700 edibles we consume today were used in prehistoric times. Even fatal poisons and their antidotes are recognized by native peoples in distant corners of this planet.

Evidence of the use of herbs as remedies 60,000 years ago during the Neanderthal period was recently uncovered by archaeologists in northern Iraq.[1] Large concentrations of the pollens of eight different medicinal plants were discovered at a human burial site there. It is unlikely they would have existed in this state without having been collected.

An Egyptian medical text dating back to between 2,600 and 2,200 B.C. lists 876 herbal prescriptions using over 500 different herbs. Recently, a Babylonian collection resembling a drug store was unearthed with an inventory of 230 herbs (first millennium B.C.). In the sixteenth century, the Spaniards reported that the Aztec herbalist had knowledge of 1,200 medicinal substances.

As one of the oldest continuous civilizations on earth, China has a long uninterrupted history of herbalism—uninterrupted in the sense that herbalism is still a very important part of everyday life today. It is routinely practiced in hospitals, clinics, and pharmacies in this country, which holds over one quarter of the Earth's population. Through thousands of years of experience, the Chinese have learned how each herb can alter and balance the energies in the body to bring about a state of health. The Chinese government has recently compiled an herbal encyclopedia that officially recognizes 5,767 medicinal herbs. The Chinese doctor prides himself on being able to prevent illness before it occurs by keeping the bodies of his patients balanced and healthy through the use of herbs as preventatives.

The Bible is also full of references pertaining to the use of herbs in healing. Revelations 22:2 says ". . . And the leaves of the tree were for the healing of the nations." In Ezekiel 47:12 the prophet advises ". . . And the fruit thereof shall be for meat, and the leaf thereof for medicine." These are only two of the biblical references stressing the importance of using herbs as medicines.

The Greeks were known to assemble this herbal knowledge and the Arabs, as traders during the Middle Ages, played an important part in spreading these understandings to other cultures. European cultures also have a long and honored history of herbalism. Great universities such as Oxford offered courses in herbal medicine until the 1700s when new chemicals were thought to be the modern way of curing the problems of the sickly. Two centuries earlier, because Henry VII was himself a bit of an herbalist, he had demanded a law to protect the right of English herbalists to practice their art.

The native peoples of America also had talented herbalists and many of their herbs were adopted by Europeans who sent the treasured medicines back to Europe. Both the native Americans and the European settlers passed the rich tradition of herbalism down from generation to generation. During the nineteenth century, herbalism was the main source of health care among most Americans. American institutions such as the Eclectic and Thompsonian herbal schools influenced the European medical movement and remained popular until the early 1940s. Even today, 25 percent of the drugs prescribed by modern doctors contain materials of plant origin. An example is the modern day aspirin, which was originally derived from the substance salicin found in white willow bark.

At one time, the effects of herbal treatments on humans and animals were a subject of intensive scientific study in the Western Hemisphere. But the development of powerful synthetic medicines (and powerful antibiotics) with the potency to annihilate dreaded diseases lured younger scientists, especially eager for new lines of study, away from botanical investigations. This was coupled with a change in the basic concept of the cause of disease. Practitioners of the old herbalism viewed disease as something wrong with the whole body, or at least a system of the body, and worked to bring about a state of health to this system through balance and nutrition. Supporters of the new beliefs, on the other hand, felt that a single disease was caused by a single pathogen that needed to be destroyed or contained.

The decline of the use of herbs can be attributed to three main factors. The first is the growth of industrialization, which took people away from the land and concentrated them in the cities. Many who harvested wild herbs now no longer had them close enough to collect conveniently. The second is the breakdown of the extended family, which made it harder for herbal knowledge to be passed along. The third is the development of synthetic pharmaceuticals and the change in scientific thinking as discussed in the previous paragraph, which brought about an acceptance of these new synthetics over the use of herbal remedies.

In even more recent times, natural healing has been ignored because it sometimes is not considered fast enough for our pace of living. In addition, since it is not always recognized as being valid by the medical institutions, some individuals do not fully trust natural treatment. Also, many people who would prefer natural treatment are not able to afford it because insurance companies do not support healing methods unless they are endorsed by licensed medical practitioners.

We shouldn't return to the era before modern medical research, but it is also a serious mistake to discard centuries of medical investigation with natural substances. Fortunately, many European scientists continued to study the health benefits of botanical preparations using the latest technologies available. References to these studies are found in the British medical reference, *The Lancet,* as well as other prominent European medical journals. To this day some herbal products outsell drugs in Europe. Ginkgo extract, for example, is used to treat a variety of ailments associated with old age, including memory loss, and is the best-selling pharmaceutical product in France and Germany.[2] Herbs contain a dramatic potency for relief, healing, cure, and prevention of disease. Modern research and technology is giving increased validity to the use of botanicals in medicine. As people assert their desire to use more natural and safer means of treating their ills, herbalism is establishing a more important role in modern health care systems.

Herbal Products Today

An important part of the art of herbal medicine is knowing what techniques to use when preparing the herbs as medicinals. The properties of an herb involve a complex synergy that acts to create a therapeutic whole from the many substances present within it. Methods of preparation have been developed over centuries to allow these properties to be released, without destroying or losing part of the healing power inherent in the herbs.

Standardized herb preparations that guarantee exact amounts of certain active ingredients combine thousands of years of herbal wisdom with the world's latest scientific research and technologies. This combination has resulted in natural, botanical products that have consistent, guaranteed activity levels. This means that you no longer need to wonder if you're getting the same strength of herb from day to day because of fluctuations in growing, harvesting, and processing methods. Scientists have confirmed that each herb, as with vitamins, has its own optimum activity level at which the best results are achieved. This means that taking less or even more than this optimum level may not give the most beneficial effects.

Until now, traditional usage has indicated a lot about how herbs can improve our health, but the actual strength of the herbs available varies so much that it is hard to rely on them completely. With standardization, however, we now know exactly what is in each tablet. Modern companies supplying standardized herbs guarantee the consistency of each tablet. Each contains the optimum activity level developed by research that, in Europe, has been going on for over fifty years. It's fortunate, that, at last, these state-of-the-art products are now available to us here in America.

In addition, some companies utilize another technological advancement known as potentization. This process is achieved by isolating the active components of the particular herb and adding more of these components back into the whole herb. The results provide a product with a strong concentration of the active ingredients giving a more powerful medicinal effect. At the same time, all naturally occurring substances are included as there is much evidence that better healing results are achieved when all parts of the herb are present than if only the active ingredients are administered.

There is another school of thought with the opinion that not only does the herb have to be complete for the best results but also all the parts need to be present in the same ratio as they are found in nature. In other words, they feel that potentization changes the make-up of the plant and therefore, a potentized product cannot demonstrate the same healing qualities as the original botanical that Mother Nature has provided. I have found extraordinary products from manufacturers that support both points of view.

One other development that has added to the quality of natural healing products is the wide range of products and information available. Due to these factors, we find some modern companies combining the herbal wisdom of both the East and West to come up with some very fine herbal concoctions. Until recently, it would have been rare to find someone educated in both Eastern and Western medicinal herbs with the supply of raw products to mix them.

So standardization, potentization, testing technologies, a wider variety of herbs, and information to work with, have all contributed to more effective products. As science continues to investigate the medicinal properties of our botanical world and continues to apply technological advancements to creating better natural products, we can expect to see more excellent natural medicines available to us.

Homeopathy

The word, homeopathy, was derived from the words *homeo* (sameness) and *pathos* (disease). Homeopathy is a therapeutic system of medicine developed by Dr. Samuel Hahnemann in Germany nearly 200 years ago. Hahnemann was a physician and biochemist who was struck by the lack of experimental support for the treatments of his day. He was inspired to establish a scientific basis for medical practice and became interested in a substance known as quinine. Jesuit missionaries brought

Peruvian bark (*cinchona*), a plant containing quinine, back to Europe from South America after they discovered the Indians were successfully treating malaria with it. Dr. Hahnemann found that when he ingested a dose of quinine, it made him feel and display the symptoms as if he had contracted malaria himself. Other investigators confirmed his findings.

Hahnemann proceeded to investigate other medicines, testing them on himself and other healthy humans, to establish precisely how they affected the human body. After some research, he concluded that symptoms are not so much a result of disease, but actually a sign of the body's resistance to disease. In 1810 he published the first edition of *Organaon of Medicine*, which set forth the basis of homeopathy in a systematic and scientific manner.

From this discovery, Hahnemann proposed the Law of Similars, the basis of homeopathic medicine. This law states that a substance given in large crude dosages will produce specific mental and physical symptoms, but when this same material has been reduced in size and administered in minute doses, it will stimulate the body's reactive processes to remove these same symptoms. One example is *ipecacuanha*, also known as ipecac root. When it is taken in large quantities, it produces vomiting, but taken in very minute doses, it cures vomiting. When administered in minute homeopathic dosages, it is even known to stop the gagging that follows coughing spells.

The holistic nature of homeopathy is best described in *Homeopathic Medicine at Home* by Panos and Heimlich:

"The homeopath believes that the body is always striving to keep itself healthy, or in balance, just as a keel boat attempts to right itself in the water. The force that acts in this protective manner is called the vital force. When the body is threatened by harmful external forces, the vital force, or defense mechanism, produces symptoms such as pain, fever, mucus, cough. These symptoms, although unpleasant for the patient, have a purpose: to restore harmony or balance. Pain is a warning that something is wrong. Fever inactivates many viruses that attack the body. Mucus is produced in the respiratory tract to surround and carry off irritating material. A cough expels the mucus that would otherwise hinder breathing."[3]

At the turn of the century, there were 22 homeopathic medical schools in the United States, over 100 homeopathic hospitals, and more than 1,000 homeopathic pharmacies. Today there are no homeopathic schools, hospitals, or pharmacies in the United States. Less than 1,000 doctors now use homeopathics in their practices compared to more than 14,000 who practiced at the turn of the century. In Europe, as with herbalism, homeopathy is much more widely accepted. France alone supports nearly 11,000 homeopathic doctors and practically every pharmacy carries homeopathic remedies.

This loss of homeopathic knowledge in U.S. medical institutions is similar to the herbal knowledge that was abandoned for new technological discoveries dealing with chemical medicines. The development of synthetic pharmaceuticals and the change in scientific thinking, which was already discussed when dealing with the history of herbal medicine, offered health practitioners the excitement of faster-acting agents to treat disease. Unfortunately, in the haste to develop these exciting new substances, the knowledge and use of the safe and useful homeopathic preparations was abandoned.

American resistance is surprising considering that schooling for a well-trained homeopath is even more extensive than for a regular medical doctor. He or she is an M.D. and needs to study everything required in a standard medical school program, plus homeopathy.[4] George Vithoulkas writes in *Homeopathy: Medicine of the New Man*, "The homeopath considers the whole body and the personality of the patient when searching for a proper treatment." This means that not only does the professional homeopath need to be familiar with over 1,000 different medicines, but he must know all the intricate and subtle signs a patient may show to determine which medicine is the proper one to administer.

The homeopath studies his patient in great detail, usually taking at least two hours for an examination. The person's physiological and psychological personality and constitution are studied in depth. Even the patient's likes and dislikes are examined. After careful consideration of the patient's symptoms and his background, he is often able to choose the remedy that is suitable for that individual.

Any substance from animal, vegetable, and mineral sources may be used in homeopathic medicines and are usually referred to as remedies. Plants are the primary source for homeopathic remedies, comprising about 80 percent of all preparations. Some examples include *Rhus toxicodendron* (poison ivy), and *Bryonia* (wild hops). Next come animal preparations such as *Apis mellifica* (honey bee) and *Sepia* (inky fluid from cuttlefish). Mineral remedies comprise the smallest category and include *Silicea* (flint) and *Natrum muriaticum* (sodium chloride or ordinary table salt) to name a few. The tiny quantities, which were discussed earlier, are prepared in a method of dilution called potentization.

Preparation of Homeopathic Remedies

Homeopathic remedies are produced either by diluting a liquid substance in distilled water, or by pounding a solid substance in a mortar along with another inert substance. The preparation is then made into its therapeutic form: either pills, powder, granules, tinctures, or ointments. The unusual thing about this process is the greater the dilution, the more powerful the substance becomes in its ability to stimulate the appropriate healing reactions.

Homeopathic remedies are prepared in decimal (log10) scales designated by the letter x, and centesimal (log100) dilutions, which may or may not be designated by the letter c. In the decimal system, one part of the material you wish to use for the basis of a remedy is mixed with nine parts of the diluent (a diluting agent such as alcohol) and shaken. Such a preparation is designated as a 1x remedy. A 2x remedy is obtained by repeating this process twice, resulting in one part to 99 parts diluent. A 3x remedy is one part to 999 parts diluent and requires repeating the diluting process three times, and so on. The centesimal is one part to 99 parts of the diluent or 1c. A 3c and a 6x remedy have the same amount of source product, but the latter has been handled and shaken twice as many times. As a general rule, beginners should use 3x, 6x, or 12x preparations.

These potentized substances stimulate the body's natural defenses to help return the patient to a state of health. These medicines will not cover up or stifle a symptom and a period of time may pass before you see a person completely restored to health. If a remedy does not cause the stimulus needed it will simply be passed off as a minute amount of natural substance. Because of this, homeopathic remedies are considered extremely safe.[5]

It is important to understand something of the delicate nature of homeopathic remedies. Because of the subtle energies that initiate healing responses in these medications, certain precautions are recommended in the handling of homeopathics to avoid contamination of the products. The lid should remain tightly sealed on the container whenever the medications are not in use. When a dose of the pellet form of a homeopathic preparation is being administered, the pellets should be gently tapped into the lid of the bottle to avoid contact with the hands. At no time should pellets be removed and then returned to the bottle, other than if they were just inside the cap of the bottle. Once the proper number of pellets are in the lid they may be slipped into the mouth, as any additional handling can contaminate the remedy, diluting its efficiency. It is said that if the pellets (or in some cases, drops) are placed under the tongue, the action of the preparation will take place more rapidly. It is also advisable when taking a homeopathic remedy to refrain from eating or drinking for fifteen minutes before or thirty minutes after ingesting a dosage. This practice allows the subtle energies present in the remedy to remain unaffected by energies in other substances. By following these guidelines you will keep the effectiveness of your homeopathic products at their peak.

We talked about the prevalence of drug side effects and, because of this risk, government agencies require that all drugs carry a written insert informing the consumer about any possible harmful reactions. Homeopathic remedies neither cover up nor cure disease by themselves. They simply stimulate the body's resources to throw off the disorder. The body's natural capacity to heal itself is safely and effectively enhanced with homeopathic medicines. Therefore, they do not create side effects and no warnings are required on homeopathic medicines beyond the usual common sense reminder: If symptoms persist or increase in severity, consult a physician.

There are products available that combine a number of remedies and thus make it easier for the untrained individual to select a specific treatment for a specific ailment. There also are homeopathic first-aid kits with a collection of common remedies complete with instructions on their use. An excellent guide to the use of homeopathics is titled *The Family Guide to Self-Medication*, which is published by the homeopathic firm Boericke & Tafel. It is advisable, however, to contact a homeopath and gain some understanding about your own body type before you attempt complex treatments yourself.

Though it is a long, extensive process to be trained as a seasoned homeopathic doctor, there are some remedies that can be helpful as first-aid items and are beneficial to have around the house. I will be mentioning some of these in the appropriate chapters. The purpose of this discussion is to give you a bit of a background and an understanding of the action of these agents. If you are interested in learning more about the science of homeopathy, an excellent resource is *The Complete Book of Homeopathy* by Dr. Michael Weiner. This comprehensive text provides an in-depth introduction to the theories and the practice of this form of holistic medicine.

Mental Influences Affecting Health

The health of our physical bodies has a direct relationship to our mental condition. Since health is such an incredible gift, we need to do all we can to insure it. This means we need to give some attention to the state of our minds as well as our physical health, because mental upset and physical disease are closely linked.

The medical community has many documented instances indicating that negative emotions have caused serious illnesses. Their concern with what is known as their "bedside manner" is evidence of a doctor's understanding of the relationship between healing and a good mental attitude. Intense grief has been known to inhibit the gastric secretions and even turn the hair white. Fear can relax the bowels and even the bladder. A fit of anger will raise the pH of the bile, raise the blood pressure, and in exaggerated cases, even turn the saliva poisonous! Sudden fright can cause violent trembling and even cardiac arrest.[6]

Hate, grief, panic, fear, despair, guilt, criticism, anger, resentment, and misery all can have a detrimental effect on your physical well-being. The old saying, "You have something on your chest," can, in effect, inhibit the natural energy flow in this part of the body and can lead to a chest or bronchial condition. People who feel like they carry a heavy burden on their shoulders often develop tight shoulder muscles. This could indicate their attitude towards responsibility should be examined.[7] A stiff neck can be a sign of inflexibility in our thinking and throat conditions are sometimes linked with the fear of self-expression.[8]

The strength of the mind is an awesome thing. In *Psycho Cybernetics*, Maxwell Maltz wrote about an experiment written up in *Research Quarterly*. Three groups of boys were selected to shoot baskets and tested for their accuracy in making their basketball free-throw shots. For twenty days, the first group practiced shooting for twenty minutes per day, the second group did no practice, and the third group sat down and imagined shooting baskets for twenty minutes per day. If this group imagined they missed a shot, he had them imagine they corrected to make the shot.

The results were quite amazing. The group that had done nothing showed no improvement, and the group that had practiced shooting baskets improved their score by 24 percent. The surprising part was that the group that had just imagined they had shot baskets showed almost as much improvement as the group that had really practiced. Their score improved 23 percent![9] Most of us have heard it stated that we only use a tiny percent of our mind's potential. How much power does our mind actually contain?

Our attitudes are definitely a factor in maintaining our physical health. When we break down the word dis-ease, we see that, by definition, a condition in our body could indicate a lack of ease mentally or emotionally. Louise L. Hay, a teacher of healing methods, firmly believes that ill health can be a reflection of a mental or emotional imbalance. In her book *Heal Your Body*, she describes her experience with using the mind to untie the knots it sometimes holds us in physically.

Louise found herself with cancer of the vagina. She believed that cancer comes from long-held resentment that literally eats at the body.[10] With a background of being raped and battered as a child, she suspected a mental pattern that developed from this time was at the bottom of her problem. Up until this point, she was unaware that she was harboring such feelings. She started working on herself with affirmations to clear these old patterns of resentment. She also worked with a nutritionist to detoxify the body. In just six months, her doctors found that there was no longer any cancer in her body.

Louise believes that both the good in our lives and the disease are a result of mental thought patterns formed from our experiences. She teaches that as long as there is a willingness to release the need we subconsciously think we have for a mental attitude, we can change these attitudes by repeating the right affirmations. In her book, she suggests different affirmations, depending on the condition, to help correct detrimental mental patterns.

Most of us are capable of shaping our destinies through the use of affirmations. Affirmations serve to recondition and re-program the mind. Because the mind is so powerful, a strong positive suggestion, if repeated often enough, can initiate a change. There are several companies that sell subliminal tapes to change behavior. These tapes repeat affirmation after affirmation masked by music and inaudible to the conscious mind. The unconscious mind, however, hears every word and after continuous exposure, can be reprogramed. Starting sentences with phrases such as, "I definitely know that" or "I am positively sure that" can produce an affirmation. For example, "I definitely know that my body will heal itself and health and well being will be a reality for me." Repeated time and time again with conviction, positive affirmations can bring about dramatic changes in our behavior and our health.

One exercise using affirmations that can be quite effective is to take a piece of colored paper and write the affirmation(s) of your choice on it. Tape the affirmation on your bathroom mirror and every morning and evening repeat it three times with as much emotion and conviction as you can muster. At the same time, take an identical piece of paper, and cut or tear it in tiny bits. Stick these tiny bits of paper to different places that you frequent regularly, for example; the refrigerator handle, the rear view mirror, or the remote for your TV. If you are doing your exercise in front of the mirror properly, your subconscious mind will repeat the affirmations every time it sees the colored bits of paper, even though you may not consciously notice them. The result is the equivalent of saying the affirmations many times during the day.

A sensitive British physician, pathologist, bacteriologist, and immunologist named Edmond Bach, who had a deep love for nature, searched for remedies that would be neither harmful nor unpleasant. He discovered a relationship between subtle energies found in plants and human emotions. After intensive research, Bach found that certain wildflowers, when picked at a certain time in their blooming cycle and prepared by a simple method, optimized the plant's healing qualities.

He taught that behind all disease lies our fears, our anxieties, our greed, our likes, and our dislikes. If we can heal these attitudes and emotions, we can heal our diseases. He felt that the mind—being the most delicate and sensitive part of the body—shows the progression of disease, and, thus, can be used to choose which remedies are necessary. Dr. Bach claimed that when we are ill, a change of mood appeared, sometimes even before the physical symptoms. For this reason he taught that an observant individual can prevent a malady from ever appearing.

Bach discovered thirty-eight different flower remedies that, when taken for specific moods, tended to "smooth out" these emotions. One of his most popular remedies is a combination of five flowers. These include: star-of-Bethlehem for shock, rock rose for terror and panic, impatiens for mental stress and tension, cherry plum for desperation, and clematis for faintness. This combination, known as "Rescue Remedy" is a great preparation for neutralizing some of the mental patterns that contribute to disease. It is often taken if one is ill, under stress, in a state of shock, or just feeling a bit out of sorts. I will speak more specifically about this remedy in future chapters.

Since Bach developed his remedies, others have expanded on his findings and developed other flower essences. Flower remedies are not chemical agents or drugs. They are liquid, potentized preparations carrying the imprint or essence of a particular flower. They are considered to be a medium that correlates the outer language of nature with inner human nature.

The remedies are taken in small dosages of 3 to 4 drops and the dosage is repeated about 3 times over a period of 15 to 30 minutes. This series can be repeated 3 or more times during the day. Many small dosages work much more effectively than one large dose. The flower essences are most effective when used in a complete health program including exercise, nourishing diet, stress reduction, appropriate medical care, and other natural therapies.

There is another subtle therapy which is being used and considered in treatment more and more. Aromatherapy is the therapeutic use of essential oils derived from plants, flowers, shrubs, and trees. The premise behind aromatherapy is that the aromas for these oils produce certain behavioral responses in the patient. For example, the herb rosemary has antiseptic and stimulating qualities and its aroma has been known to help with headaches, colds, bronchitis, and muscular pains.[11] Aromatherapy oils can be added to bath water, massage oils, or simply inhaled to produce their effects. Healing results produced by different aromas may include calming, stimulating, centering, or some other beneficial effect.

The point to be stressed here is that our mental well being, or the lack of it, can have a striking effect on our physical health. Because the mind is such a powerful tool, it would benefit us to have a healthy, loving outlook when we are trying to heal ourselves or we simply want to stay healthy. You can use some of the tools I have mentioned or whatever means you find work best for you. Regardless of our physical health, life is a much more enjoyable experience when our minds are at ease.

Bodywork and Energy Balancing

When you are experiencing discomfort from illness, injury, or just aches and pains, you might find a session with a good bodywork specialist to be just what you need. Often, aches or illnesses are simply a result of the stress in our daily lives. These discomforts may be a result of external factors such as a stressful work environment or, as mentioned previously, from internally generated mental or emotional tension. Regardless of the cause, a good therapist trained in bodywork techniques may be just what you need.

Bodywork, for those not familiar with the term, refers to a number of different techniques that include working on someone's body with the hands. This "hands-on" work can be gentle and soothing or intense and stimulating, and can work to manipulate the muscle tissue and/or to stimulate and move body energy.

There are many schools of thought governing the techniques used in bodywork systems. Often one system will benefit a particular individual while another will not be quite right, just as one doctor may be right for one while not adequate for another. Also, the nature of the healing need of the patient will vary and be a factor in determining the bodywork practitioner a person chooses.

Touch can be a very effective means of healing. The simple act of caring for someone through the medium of touch and massage can do wonders for a person's self-acceptance. When a person is feeling discomfort, it is helpful to have the support of someone knowledgeable who can assist him or her with their quest for health. Touching, given with tenderness and care, can cause wonderful transformations both physically and psychologically. When properly done, massage relaxes the body, increases circulation and sensation, and promotes a sense of well being.

You may want to go to a bodywork specialist because you are experiencing some physical pain or because you are simply feeling tightness in your muscles due to tension or stress. A good massage therapist will manipulate and massage the muscles to work out the "knots" of tension, leaving the body in a relaxed condition.

There are many different types of massage. Because of the wide range of techniques, they are far too numerous to list here completely. I will, however, briefly mention a few of the more popular types. Please understand that I will be giving you a very tiny glimpse of each one and the only way to gain any real understanding as to what each system encompasses is to find a qualified practitioner and experience a session for yourself. I can think of fewer things more pleasant than experiencing an assortment of different massage techniques.

One very popular massage method is called Swedish massage. The therapist massages one area of muscles after another until the entire body has been worked. In Swedish massage, the therapist massages each muscle until its stored tension literally melts away. This leaves the individual who received the massage in a wonderful state of relaxation.

Sports massage is aimed at treating sports injuries. Often, sports teams will have a full-time practitioner experienced in sports-massage techniques at every game and practice. These therapists have a keen knowledge of the body, how muscles and other connective tissues work, and many techniques to help the healing process in case of injury.

Other methods, including rolfing and similar systems, use extremely deep pressure in specific points and areas of the body in order to correct the structure of the connection tissue. Rolfing enthusiasts claim that their deep pressure techniques actually realign the body. Once aligned and balanced, the body interacts with gravity to achieve graceful movement and a free flow of energy.[12] Some people report that they are taller after a series of rolfing sessions because their spines have been straightened and that negative emotional patterns locked in the body have been released. Because of the deep work that is involved, rolfing and similar therapies can be a bit painful.

Another science of structural bodywork that many people are familiar with is chiropractic medicine. The basic principle of chiropractic is that the human body, with its nervous system working at its full potential, is capable of maintaining perfect health. Since the spinal column is the life line of the nervous system, it needs to be cared for and maintained to benefit balance in the entire body.[13] This is accomplished through a series of manipulations on the spine resulting in all the vertebrae (spinal bones) lining up in their proper positions. It often takes a series of adjustments, depending on how serious the condition is, before the out-of-line vertebrae will remain in their proper places.

Though any time you massage or manipulate areas of the body you will tend to move energy around; certain systems of bodywork were developed specifically for this purpose. Specific channels of energy help to regulate corresponding organs, actions, or processes in the body. By stimulating specific points, a knowledgeable person can cause energy to flow, achieving particular results. The movement of energy will often release accumulated toxins. These accumulations cause blocks that inhibit the energy to flow as it would under normal, healthy conditions.

There are several different systems that utilize the techniques of energy stimulation. Shiatsu and acupressure tend to work on specific points in the body related to different organs and other body parts that need special attention. Shiatsu massage is derived from traditional Japanese finger pressure massage. It involves dispersing of excess or blocked energy through slow, deep penetration of key points along the acupuncture meridians. Acupuncture meridians are recognized channels of energy related to functions in the body. Acupressure massage, a similar Chinese healing art, is related to acupuncture, except that, instead of using needles to stimulate specific points, the hands are used. Another modern day healing system derived from the ancient acupressure, is reflexology. In reflexology, points in the hands and feet are stimulated to increase energy flow and cleanse related parts of the body.

Still another healing science is polarity therapy, which works with the electromagnetic energy in the body. This subtle system of energy patterns has an effect when in balance, that contributes to the body's natural state of health. Basically, it is the science of balancing the life energy in the human body. When that energy is balanced on all levels, we experience a state of health. The therapist accomplishes this balance by holding two points on the body while utilizing certain polarity principles as developed by its founder, Dr. Randolph Stone. By repeating this process on different combinations of points, he is able to clear and balance particular energies and allow the subject's energy to flow as it naturally should. Polarity is a holistic system in that it utilizes diet, exercise, manipulation, and mental attitude to achieve optimal wellness.

Many excellent therapists use a combination of techniques from a number of these and other disciplines. In this way they are able to work on a range of different problems in a variety of different ways. Bodywork often requires trusting your intuitive nature to guide you with your choices of techniques and methods. As mentioned before, certain techniques may be appropriate in one situation and not in another.

I included this discussion of bodywork principles for three reasons. The first, since this book is concerned with tools that help the body in its quest for health, was to make you aware of another realm of natural healing tools, the methods found in the bodywork field. I hope I have given you a brief introduction into this varied and valuable science. The second reason I included this subject was because I wanted to share some simple techniques as tools for a specific purpose in later chapters of this writing. And the third and perhaps most important reason was to mention the importance of energy and balance.

There is a certain intelligence to the energy I speak of that somehow knows how to keep or restore health to a body almost regardless of what abuse we inflict upon ourselves. When this energy is allowed to flow unhindered by toxins, emotions, mental attitudes, or injuries, health is a natural occurrence. This occurs when we experience balance.

Balance in one's life, I feel, is essential to health. According to *Dorland's Medical Dictionary*, health is "a state of complete physical, mental, and social well-being, and not merely the absence of disease and infirmity." In other words, only when we are in balance in every way, can we claim we are healthy. Behind and within everything, whether it is a medicine, an herb, a food, or within a human being's emotions, mental state, or physical condition, there are exact qualities of energy. When these emotional, mental, and physical states are brought into balance, either through the balancing forces of bodywork techniques or with the help of foods or medicines (also expressions of energy that contribute to balance), we experience health. More accurately, the energies in the foods and medicines we ingest help stimulate our body's own mechanisms capable of restoring balance and health to the whole being. This energy, this intelligence inherent in us all, is the real healer. All the therapists, techniques, healthful foods, and medicines merely assist this energy to do its work unhindered.

3

Eating Right

Health is such a wonderful gift that one should do whatever is within one's power to secure it. Unfortunately, most people do not think too seriously about their health until it begins to slip away. Much too little attention is given to the preservation of health. One of the goals of holistic medicine is to enable us to retain our sound constitutions. There are so many foods within our reach these days and it's left up to each one of us to choose the menus that will contribute to our long-term well being. Though it is hard to resist many of the succulent treats available that could cause unfortunate results for our bodies, we should use our common sense and not overindulge our cravings for poor food. Did you know that some experts have estimated that as many as 35 percent of cancer deaths are diet-related? We often lose sight of the purpose of food and may want to ask ourselves the question, "Do we live to eat or eat to live?"

When all cells, tissues, glands, and organs are working harmoniously and optimally together, we might consider ourselves to be in a true state of health. In other words, a state of perfect health may be a long distance from being "sick." Many conditions such as sweet cravings, low energy, irritability, allergies, having an excess of gas, susceptibility to cold, and other minor conditions that may be overlooked, can be symptoms of health problems. Optimally functioning systems of immunity, excretion, digestion, circulation, endocrine secretions, and nervous responses are all necessary for the body to resist disease-causing agents before they can create enough damage to result in bodily ills.

As mentioned before, I am not preaching total abstinence from foods known to be unhealthy. In most cases, all that's needed is some common-sense moderation. You really needn't live a boring life to remain healthy. You can structure the majority of your diet with good foods, most of which can be prepared quite deliciously by the way, and help your body in the battle to maintain a healthy state in the midst of a modern lifestyle.

What Is Healthy Eating?

Depending on whom you consult, healthy eating can have many different meanings. The macrobiotic diet consists mostly of heavily cooked grains and vegetables. On the other hand, raw food enthusiasts claim that it is unhealthy to eat cooked food. They maintain that most of the nutritive value is destroyed when a food is heated beyond a certain temperature. Many of us learned in grade school that a balanced meal must include meat to insure the proper amount of protein. But we have since learned that there are plenty of strong, healthy vegetarians walking around. The more you read about "healthy diets," the more confused you can become!

One common misconception is that the diet that improves your health will continue to support your health over a long period of time. For instance, an unhealthy person becomes healthy after sticking to a strict regime of raw fruit and fruit juice. He then decides that this is the healthy way to eat and continues to follow the diet for an extended period of time. Now some individuals may do fine on fruit for long periods of time, but chances are that most people will find themselves severely out-of-balance on such a severe diet. The point is that foods can be medicines and can bring an unbalanced condition into balance, but they can also cause an imbalance if overdone. If you are instructed to take a medicine to cure an illness, when you are cured you should discontinue the regime. The same is true when using diet to cure conditions. This doesn't mean you need to go back to the poor diet you indulged in that made you ill in the first place. Just learn how to be balanced in what you eat and always to use good judgement. Remember: The cure is not always the rule, and the rule is not always the cure!

However, there are some points that many health experts agree on in regards to good dietary standards and I will list a few of them here. If we know the general rules, then all we need to do is to make sure we try to eat most of the foods that will nourish us. There is one thing in our favor anyway. Nowadays, there are more and more very tasty substitutions for some of the junk food we've grown to love.

Eating Habits

Eating too much at a meal is an important habit to avoid. Overeating, even of healthy foods, is not much better than eating unhealthy foods. Not only is there a tendency towards unnecessary weight gain, but the body feels sluggish and the mind, in turn, slows down. Snacking is often the biggest culprit contributing to overeating. Try to eliminate this nasty habit by sticking to a strict schedule of eating only at mealtimes. This procedure may need to be adapted for some people, especially those who suffer from hypoglycemia (low blood sugar). For these individuals, a regime of five meals (three medium-sized and two small) may work better to maintain proper blood sugar levels. When I speak of snacking, I'm referring to that unnecessary bag of chips and handful of cookies we often grab between meals, usually due to poor eating habits.

Sometimes, overeating can signify a craving for something you are missing nutritionally or even emotionally. Often, people will overeat when they try to quit smoking or when they split up with a lover or spouse. Try to get in touch with your feelings if you're stuffing yourself as a result of an emotional crisis. In some cases, professional counseling may be helpful. If a nutritional deficiency is causing your cravings, a nutritionist may be able to help you find the vitamin or mineral you lack.

It is important to not eat your food too quickly. Slow eating and efficient mastication are essential for proper health. Eating too fast really short circuits the digestive machine. The mouth is a primary organ of digestion. The enzyme *ptyalin*, found in the saliva, is necessary for the breakdown of carbohydrates. The action of this enzyme allows well-chewed food to be half digested by the time it gets to the stomach. If your food is not allowed to be broken down by chewing and these enzymes are not able to mix with the food adequately, it may putrefy in the digestive tract and cause flatulence (commonly known as gas). Much of the nutritive value of the food will be lost as well, because the food will not have been made available for easy absorption by the body.

Eating slower will help you with overeating as well. If we eat too fast, we often eat past the point of being stuffed. Eating slowly allows a little time for the stomach to let the brain know when we've reached our limit.

The most preferred methods of cooking foods are steaming, baking, broiling, and lightly sautéing under low to medium heat. When steaming, many of the nutrients are leached into the water, which can later be used for a nutritious soup stock. When sautéing, if the oil becomes too hot, it becomes rancid and difficult to digest. Adding a bit of water to the vegetables will cook them faster and allow the temperature to remain lower. The best oils to use when sautéing include butter, virgin olive oil, canola, sesame, high-oleic safflower or high-oleic sunflower. These oils are better for sautéing because they contain less saturated fats and/or because they tend not to break down as easily as other oils when heated at high temperatures.

Avoid using aluminum pots and pans as the aluminum that leaches into the food can be poisonous. Enamel cookware is usually aluminum underneath an enamel coating, which tends to scratch or chip allowing the aluminum to leach through. Not sharing this problem, stainless steel, glass, and cast iron cookware are good alternatives to aluminum.

Processed Foods

It's a good idea to eliminate processed foods from your diet as much as is possible. Sometimes refined foods are not necessarily "bad" for you; they just don't provide many of the vitamins and minerals that a healthy body needs. If a large part of your diet is composed of overly refined foods such as white bread and white rice, and you are not in the habit of taking plenty of supplements, you may be starving yourself of some necessary nutrients. To make white flour, the outer skin known as the "bran" and the living part known as the "germ" are both removed. What is left is mostly starch. Most of the real nutritional value is found in these other two elements, and though the starch is also something the body needs to operate properly, it doesn't provide everything necessary for health.

On the other hand, many heavily processed foods can be much more detrimental to our health. Sugar is becoming more and more well known as the culprit leading to various health disorders. I once had a friend who worked in a sugar processing plant. He told me that the raw sugar beets went through several floors of a building the length of a long city block, with many chemicals added in the processing. His job was to pour a bucket of formaldehyde into the sugar beet pulp at his position in the processing line. Some people know the mortician's name for formaldehyde: embalming fluid!

Whole grains and whole foods are really delicious and can easily be substituted for processed foods. Whole wheat bread, whole grain brown rice, and natural sugar substitutes such as fruit-juice sweetener, rice syrup, malt syrup, sucanat (pure cane juice), maple syrup, and honey are all better choices as sweeteners as they contain more nutrition in the form of vitamins and minerals. Whenever possible, substitute fresh or frozen fruits and vegetables for overly cooked canned products. Because of the superior food value in these products, you will be getting a lot more for your money.

I needn't go into detail about the detrimental effects of the over-use of alcohol, nicotine, caffeine, or recreational drugs. By now, everyone is aware that our bodies can only stand so much abuse from such substances. As you begin to eat a better diet, you will become more conscious and sensitive to the types of foods your body prefers and start to respond to its signals. If you partake in any of these substances, you should observe extreme moderation, for it is the nature of these subtle poisons to slowly degenerate one of your most precious possessions— your health.

If a dependence has developed for any of these substances, it can be caused by nutritional imbalances. Researchers have recently discovered that the brains of alcoholics produce THIQ, a particular chemical that seems to contribute to alcoholism.[1] These findings indicate that genetic factors may make some individuals more prone to addictive behavior. An excellent resource if you or someone you love is affected by an addictive disease is the book by John Finnegan *Addictions, A Nutritional Approach to Recovery.* This helpful guide outlines metabolic causes of addictions and practical therapies to correct these biochemical disorders.

Food Additives

Avoid food additives and preservatives! Many highly questionable chemicals are added to foods either to preserve, to keep from separating, to facilitate preparation, to color, to flavor, or to otherwise enhance consumer acceptability of the product. Food processors have an estimated 10,000 chemicals they can add to what we eat. Some are beneficial, some are harmless, and some are poisonous. Some 200 different "standard" food products, including mayonnaise, catsup, and ice cream are not even required to list all their ingredients. The manufacturer is able to choose among many standard chemicals and need only list items on his product label if they are not in this category.[2]

According to Samuel Epstein, M.D., in his book *The Politics of Cancer*, "The average American eats nine pounds of chemical additives a year, including preservatives, flavoring agents, stabilizers, and artificial colors."[3] Consider what this means when extended over a few decades, much less a lifetime, and what effect these hundreds of pounds of additives can have on one's health.

It is amazing what you can find by just reading the labels of the foods not on the "standard" food list. One well-known "natural" orange-flavored drink is made up of sugar, citric acid, natural flavor, gum arabic, monosodium phosphate, potassium citrate, calcium phosphate, Vitamin C, cellulose gum, hydrogenated coconut oil, artificial flavor, artificial coloring, Vitamin A, and butylated hydroxyanisole. Another product, a whipped topping, consists of sodium caseinate, dextrose, corn sugar, polysorbate 60, sorbiyan monostearate, carageenan, and guar gum.[4] Really not too appetizing if you ask me! How many of us can read a label like this and really understand what we are consuming?

The late Will Rogers once said, "If you can't spell it, it won't work." This quote could have been made to describe food additives. I really don't feel at ease looking at a food label bearing one or more unfamiliar words with ten to twenty letters or more. An example is sulfating agents like sulfur dioxide and sodium bisulfite, which prevent discoloration in salads and dried fruits and prevent bacterial growth in wines. These products are known to have caused at least five deaths![5] Some of these chemical names are so long that they are abbreviated as in the case of butylated hydroxyanisole (BHA). In a Japanese study BHA was shown to cause cancer in rats![6] About 80 million pounds of monosodium glutamate (MSG) will be imported this year into the United States to be used as flavor enhancers. You may be familiar with a condition called "Chinese restaurant syndrome." This refers to the tightness in the chest and headache many people experience after eating an Oriental meal heavily laden with MSG. This commonly used additive has been found to cause deep depression and life-threatening asthmatic attacks in sensitive human beings. Testing has also shown MSG to cause brain damage in rats, rabbits, chicks, and monkeys.[7]

The truth is, it takes a biochemist to understand what most of these additives are. Why? Because most of these substances were created in the laboratory and do not have much in common with naturally occurring food products. In addition, many of these chemicals have been around for only a few decades and even the biochemists haven't really seen the long-range results of a diet high in these man-made substances.

Some food additives destroy or inactivate enzymes in the foods so that spoilage will not occur. It's hard to believe that, once inside the human body, these same chemicals will have absolutely no effect on the enzymes in our tissues that are so important for bodily functions. Additives are perhaps the primary factor that make junk food live up to its name. Some additives are only harmful to infants, some are more detrimental to those with food allergies, and some are bad for all of us. The more additives we consume, the greater the risk factor involved. By eating high quality, unprocessed natural foods, you won't have to worry about the possible problems that food additives may produce.

In short, be kind to your body. Check labels carefully to make sure only natural ingredients are being used in the foods you eat. Advice from Bonnie Liebman, a nutritionist for the Center for Science in the Public Interest (CSPI) suggests you should "Treat each label as if it were a contract. Read it very carefully, and look for any tricks in the fine print."[8]

Sugar

Beware of sugar! We are born into this world with a natural craving for sweets. It is nature's way of assuring we will seek out the sweet breast milk of our mothers to ensure our survival. So strong is this instinct that even an unborn fetus will make swallowing motions when its mother is injected with a sweetener. No other taste sensation will cause this impulse.[9]

Unfortunately, this normal desire for sweets can easily lead to an exaggerated and harmful habit. White sugar is two-and-a-half times sweeter than the lactose in mother's milk, and quite often an infant will reject breast milk for sweetened formulas. In our teenage years, our desire for sweets is at its highest and usually this habit is set in place for life.

Carbohydrates in the form of sugars and starches are essential to the human diet. However, refined sugar was virtually unknown to us until the fifteenth century. Up to that time, almost all sugar was consumed in the form of whole grains, fruits, and vegetables. Today, the average intake of cane and beet sugar for a U.S. citizen is estimated at approximately one-third pound per day or 125 pounds per year. This is an extremely high figure considering the health risks that are at stake.

We all know of the dental bills we can attribute to sugar. *Streptococcus mutans* is the bacteria in our mouths that feeds on sugar deposits and causes plaque. This process causes the acidity in the mouth to increase to about 100 times the normal amount, making the environment perfect for tooth decay.[10] You would think that just the desire to stay away from the dental drill would be enough to convince people to be more sensible about their intake of sweets! I find it interesting that in native cultures, which consume large amounts of raw sugar cane but no refined sugar, there is little incidence of tooth decay.

Unfortunately, tooth decay is only one of the risks taken when we succumb to our sugar cravings. Diabetes, hypoglycemia, obesity, bowel cancer, coronary thrombosis, arteriosclerosis, appendicitis, acne, schizophrenia, and other ailments are suspected to be related to excessive sugar intake.[11] With all the warnings by health professionals advising people to cut down on sweets, it is really amazing that so much sugar is still being eaten. This may substantiate the fact that many Americans are considered to be addicted to sugar. In John Finnegan's book *Addictions, A Nutritional Approach to Recovery*, he states, "Sugar is the foremost addictive substance used today and several other drugs cause highs through a similar metabolic process. Alcohol is a simple sugar. Caffeine, hallucinogens, amphetamines, and cocaine all temporarily increase the release of sugar into the bloodstream and nervous system."[12]

A refined sugar is one that is separated from the other substances found in its natural plant form. Sucrose or white sugar is the most commonly used sweetener. This is probably the worst form of sugar to consume because it has no food value except for burnable calories. White sugar contains no vitamins, minerals, or proteins. Also, it's so concentrated that it tends to send our blood sugar level to a quick peak. Our body responds to remove the excess sugar from our bloodstream by secreting added insulin. The short-term results of excess sugar and the corresponding increased level of insulin in our bodies causes our energy levels to drop to the opposite low extreme. Quite often, this drop may be accompanied by feelings of depression as well. The long-term results are wear and tear on the insulin-secreting organ, the pancreas, and perhaps the development of a hypoglycemic or a diabetic condition.

A high dietary sugar intake can cause many symptoms that we might not think to associate with our sweet tooths. Some possible symptoms of excessive sugar intake include nervousness, irritability, exhaustion, faintness, dizziness, tremors, cold sweats, depression, headaches, digestive disturbances, insomnia, cravings (for sugar and alcohol), mood swings, anxieties, mental confusion, internal trembling, rapid pulse, constant worrying, and frequent sighing and yawning.[13]

Even though eating too much of any sugar can cause health problems, some sugars contain more minerals, vitamins, and proteins than others. For instance, chromium is a trace element necessary for the metabolism of sugar. This nutrient helps insulin to work better at the cellular level. If insufficient chromium is present in the foods you are eating, the liver will be robbed of chromium to metabolize the sugar. The more a sugar is refined, the less chance it will contain essential nutrients like chromium.

Some sweeteners that contain more trace nutrients than refined sugars include honey, fruit-juice sweetener, rice syrup,
maple syrup, blackstrap molasses, sucanat (pure cane juice)
and 100 percent malt syrup. It is interesting that pure sugar
cane juice has been used for centuries by native cultures without the negative effects of white sugar.[14] If malt syrup does not
indicate it is 100 percent malt, it is probably mostly corn syrup.
Corn syrup is made up of glucose, a sweeter sugar than the
maltose in barley malt. Many people consider brown sugar to
be a healthy food. Brown sugar is no more than white sugar
with some added molasses and flavorings! It is important to
keep in mind that even preferred forms of sweeteners are still
types of concentrated sugars and over-consumption could lead
to serious health problems.

The best sources are starches because the body changes the
starches to sugars and assimilates them more slowly than refined sugars. This process of sugars entering the blood stream
slower is much gentler on our system. Also, whole foods give a
more sustained source of energy to the body instead of the
sharp swings in blood sugar levels from foods with refined
sugars.

Some people use a sugar substitute called *saccharin* to avoid
the high calories of sugar. Saccharin is 350 times sweeter than
white sugar and studies have shown that it can help people to
lose weight. Unfortunately, other studies indicate that it may
cause cancer. In 1977, the Food and Drug Administration even
proposed that saccharin be banned. It is gradually being replaced by *aspartame* (NutraSweet) and though it appears to be a
harmless product, I have yet to see the long-range effects to determine how safe NutraSweet really is.

There is a sweetening agent that is a plant extract, used for
centuries in South America and more recently in Japan, which
appears to be a safe alternative to sugar and is forty times
sweeter! This extract of the stevia plant has been subjected to
extensive research by the Japanese for safety and effectiveness.
A few drops will sweeten a cup of tea at 1/300th the calories of
the amount of white sugar it would take to do the job. In addition, it has been shown to promote mental alertness, normalize
blood sugar, lower blood pressure, aid in digestion, and even
help fight tooth decay.[15]

How much sugar should we eat? The Surgeon General's August 1988 report suggested we cut our intake of refined sugars. The government-generated goals also suggest eating less of all types of sugar and sugar-containing foods. This is generally a very attractive group of foods and not always easy for an individual to resist. Candy, cookies, cakes, sodas, and other delectable goodies top this list. The best policy is to have respect for these items and enjoy them in moderation.

Read your labels and avoid foods containing sugar that don't really need to have this ingredient included. For example, there are many delicious brands of peanut butter available that don't contain sugar, yet some companies insist on putting this ingredient in their product. Because most of us are addicted to sugar, the manufacturers are feeding this addiction to insure repeated sales of their products. If you take the time, you can also find fruit juices, canned fruit and vegetables, and other delicious products that don't contain added sugar to make them appealing. Manufacturers are required to list ingredients in order of highest concentration. If a form of sugar is one of the first ingredients listed, you can be sure there is a high concentration of sugar in the product. So watch for and avoid first ingredients (or a listing with several ingredients) labeled sucrose, dextrose, fructose, lactose, maltose, corn syrup, honey, sweeteners, or natural sweeteners. Lastly, when you do indulge in a tasty sweet treat, savor it and be moderate in your consumption.

Fats

As with proteins and carbohydrates, fats are essential elements of bodily nourishment. Fats are concentrated, energy-producing food substances. When oxidized, they provide twice as much energy as proteins and carbohydrates. They also must be present in order for Vitamins A, D, E, and K to be absorbed in the blood.[16] The only element in the body more abundant than fat is water. Seventy percent of our brain and nerve cells are made of fat as well as 30 percent of our cell membranes. Healthy cell membranes are essential if we want our cells protected from bacterial and viral invasions. Some of the benefits of a healthy nervous system include proper functioning of the musculature for normal movement and the appropriate responses by our glandular systems to properly regulate the many internal functions of the body. A normally functioning nervous system also contributes to our ability to experience a feeling of well being.

Of course, excessive fat consumption can be detrimental to our health. Some of the possible problems associated with over-consumption of fats include obesity, sugar intolerance, food sensitivities and allergies, gastrointestinal problems, liver function imbalance, endocrine imbalance, increased risk of heart disease, and increased chance of certain cancers.[17]

Recently, a study was published in the *Journal of the American Medical Association*. Based on research studying 11,864 people between the ages of 20 and 74, the researchers estimated that 36 percent of all adults in that age range (60 million people overall!) had cholesterol levels warranting medical advice and intervention. "Even though we've made great progress in preventing heart disease, cholesterol is still a serious problem in the U.S.," says Christopher Sempos of the National Center for Health Statistics. According to National Cholesterol Education Program guidelines, levels under 200 are considered good; over 240, cause for concern; between 200 and 240, a potential problem if there are at least two other risk factors.[18]

In general, Americans eat about twice as much fat as they should. Approximately 40 percent of the calories ingested are in the form of fats. Former Surgeon General Koop suggests that we reduce this rate to 30 percent. But Udo Erasmus, in his comprehensive book, *Fats & Oils*, suggests staying closer to 20 percent, saying that this would greatly reduce heart disease, cancer, and other degenerative diseases.

There are about two dozen types of fats utilized by the tissues and all but two can be synthesized by the body. These two (linoleic acid and linolenic acid) are called essential fatty acids or EFAs and are absolutely necessary for the maintenance of health. EFAs strengthen the immune system; nourish the skin, hair, nerves, thyroid, mucous membranes, and glandular systems; and aid in the prevention of arteriosclerosis and the reduction of cholesterol. EFAs are also used by our body cells for energy production.[19] All other fatty acids can be produced in the body from just these two EFAs![20]

There are both good fats and bad fats. Jeffrey Bland, Ph.D., another nutritional expert, defines good fats as those low in saturated fats with minimum processing, comparable to those our ancestors used. He defines bad fats as saturated animal and vegetable fats and unsaturated vegetable fats modified by modern processing such as hydrogenated fats.[21] Erasmus goes on to recommend unrefined oils, those which are expeller pressed (pressed at lower heat without the use of solvents such as hexane), as the preferred oils for human use. Hexane is a petroleum derivative that is known to be a mild central nervous system depressant and may also be irritating to the respiratory tract.[22]

Proper storage of your oils is also important. Store your vegetable oils away from heat, light, and air (ideally, keep oil in your refrigerator with the cap on tight) to maintain their beneficial qualities and avoid rancidity. The rancidity process in oils starts at the time the oils are made. When the oils are exposed to oxygen, they take up the oxygen molecules to form peroxides. The oxidation process speeds up as these substances are formed. Once peroxides begin to be made, they continue to form even if not exposed to oxygen.

One unsettling fact is that light causes free radical damage to oils and that light oxidation is 1,000 times faster than oxygen oxidation![23] For this reason some progressive companies are considering bottling their oils in special black plastic containers. These containers keep all the light out (some light can penetrate dark glass bottles) and have been proven to allow no transmigration of potentially carcinogenic hydrocarbons from the plastic into the oil.[24] Some companies are already doing this with a few specialized oils.

Besides altering the flavor and odor of the oils, rancidity can have detrimental effects on the body. Eating rancid oils destroys Vitamins A, E, and F stored in the body, causing deficiencies of these nutrients. Our bodies cannot properly digest or assimilate rancid oils either. It has been shown that they can irritate stomach and bowel linings and can contribute to various disorders, including cancer.

One thing you can do to improve the quality of the fats you eat is to stay away from the oils that are highest in saturated fats. Saturated fats trigger the body to produce cholesterol and can be more dangerous than eating foods containing cholesterol. All oils contain both saturated and unsaturated fats, the most desirable oils being the ones with the lowest levels of saturates. Canola, safflower, and sunflower oils contain the lowest amount of saturated fats of the commonly used vegetable oils. Canola oil contains only 6 percent saturated fats, and safflower and sunflower oils consist of 8 percent saturates.

Palm, palm kernel, and coconut oils have the highest levels of saturates of the common edible oils and are widely used because of their economical price. This price differential is due to the low cost of labor in the countries where these tropical oils are processed. Palm oil contains 86 percent saturated fats and coconut oil contains 92 percent. Most other edible oils have a saturated content of less than 20 percent. Other oils to avoid are cottonseed oil, because there is a possibility of a high pesticide content, and any hydrogenated oils.

Hydrogenated oils are produced by adding hydrogen ions to a liquid oil in order to make the oil more solid. An example is the making of margarine from a vegetable oil. Unfortunately, this process produces a substance very similar to a saturated fat. Beware of products with labels stating "cholesterol-free" while containing highly saturated or hydrogenated oils that stimulate our bodies to produce cholesterol! Another process of modern technology, homogenization, has also been shown to damage the composition of fats. This process, used to extend the shelf life of milk and other products, carries a destructive enzyme into the bloodstream that can cause damage to the arteries.[25]

Is there such a thing as a "good" fat? Yes. Cholesterols are never found free floating in the bloodstream, but are wrapped around lipoproteins (literally, fatty proteins). The "bad" cholesterols, known as low-density and very-low-density lipoproteins (LDLs and VLDLs), only carry incoming fat and cholesterol from the liver into the circulatory system, in effect, increasing cholesterol levels. The "good" cholesterols, or high-density lipoproteins (HDLs), on the other hand, actually pick up cholesterol from your arterial walls and transport it to the liver where it is broken down and flushed from the body. More scientists are becoming convinced, in fact, that the ratio of good to bad cholesterol is more relevant to heart-disease risk than overall cholesterol levels.[26]

Jane Brody, author of the best-seller *Jane Brody's Nutrition Book*, wrote in her *New York Times* health column in 1985 that monounsaturated oils "may be more helpful than polyunsaturates in preventing heart disease." Brody referred to clinical research by Dr. Scott Grundy, which indicated that while polyunsaturated fats reduced cholesterol, monounsaturated fats removed more "bad"—LDL—cholesterol than polyunsaturates. The superiority of monounsaturated oils is that they leave the blood with more "good" HDLs.[27] One indication of relationship is the low incidence of coronary heart disease in the Mediterranean region, where olive oil (a monounsaturate) has been consumed in large quantities for centuries. We'll discuss this more in the section on heart disease and nutrition. Table 3.1 gives the relative fat content of some common oils.

At the time of this writing, Congressman Dan Glickman had introduced a bill requiring all processed foods containing coconut, palm, and palm kernel oil to include the phrase, "a saturated fat." Those products stating "made with 100 percent vegetable shortening" would have to indicate which, if any, tropical oils were used and identify them as saturated fats. Labels would have to specify which oils were used in a food product instead of stating, "containing any one or more of the following."

Recently, wealthy Omaha industrialist, heart attack victim, and cholesterol crusader Phil Sokolof blasted large corporations for using these controversial oils in their products. In his ad campaign entitled "The Poisoning of America," Sokolof ran full page ads in *USA Today* and *The Wall Street Journal*. Borden, General Mills, Quaker Oats, Pillsbury, and Ralston Purina products were all named as containing tropical oils. Many of the companies claimed on their labels that their products reduced cholesterol because they contained oat bran. What they failed to mention was these same products contained oils high in saturated fats, which trigger the body to produce cholesterol. The unaware consumer who buys the product to lower cholesterol intake actually adds to his cholesterol problems. Soon after Sokolof's ad campaign, all these companies announced they had taken steps to reformulate their products. In addition Kellogg's, Nabisco, and Sunshine have been on Soko-

Table 3.1 **Fat Content of Oils**

Type of Oil	Mono- Unsaturated	Poly- Unsaturated	Saturated
Butterfat	30%	4%	66%
Canola	60%	34%	6%
Coconut	6%	2%	92%
Corn	29%	54%	17%
Cottonseed*	19%	54%	27%
Lard	47%	12%	41%
Olive	82%	8%	10%
Palm Kernel	16%	1%	83%
Peanut	60%	22%	18%
Safflower, High-Oleic	75%	17%	8%
Safflower, Regular	13%	79%	8%
Sesame	46%	41%	13%
Soy	28%	58%	14%
Sunflower	26%	66%	8%

*Be careful—Pesticide restrictions on cotton are not as stringent as on other oil crops.

lof's hit list, and these companies are apparently also making efforts to improve the oils in their product lines.

Unfortunately, these tropical oils were often replaced with hydrogenated soybean oils and, if this is the case, no real improvement has been made. Wouldn't it be great if concern for their customers' welfare was genuine enough to these large food corporations that they actually decided to improve the quality of the oils in all their products as well as improve any other questionable ingredients?

Salt

Salt, or sodium chloride, is a necessary component of the human diet. It is needed for different metabolic functions including the production of hydrochloric acid in the stomach. A person needs from 0.2 to 0.6 grams (1/25th to 1/8th teaspoon) of salt per day, which can easily be obtained from a diet containing plenty of raw foods. Raw foods are required because cooking often removes much of the salt and other minerals from foods. Most Americans use way too much salt, as much as 10 to 15 grams every day. At four times the world's average, salt is so prevalent in the American diet that simply by reducing one's intake by not adding any salt at all to meals, Americans would still get about two-thirds of needed daily intake hidden in prepared and processed foods.[28]

The kidneys are capable of removing up to five grams of sodium chloride per day. A recent study conducted on two groups of rats, one with a high-salt diet and one with a low-salt diet, showed that in a stressful environment the rats that ate the high-salt diet retained much of the salt in their systems.[29] Excess salt stays in the body and is stored in various organs and tissues. Too much salt can cause many problems, including high blood pressure, heart and circulatory system conditions, kidney disorders, hair loss, and skin problems. Edema is usually an indication that there is excess salt being stored in the tissues due to an overworked kidney.[30]

One of the first effective treatments for hypertension (high blood pressure) was to reduce salt intake. As antihypertensive drugs and diuretics were developed, sodium restriction was considered less important. Now that there is concern about side effects of such drug treatment, non-drug alternatives are being investigated with renewed interest. In fact, researchers at the Einstein Medical College of Yeshiva University in New York City conclude that drastic lowering of blood pressure with drugs actually increases the risk of heart attacks.[31] Recent research has shown that reducing salt intake moderately can produce a significant decrease in blood pressure. A 30-day study involving 114 patients on hypertensive medication showed that a low-salt diet not only reduced blood pressure in 30.4 percent of the subjects, but allowed many of the subjects to reduce their medication levels as well.[32]

There is also scientific evidence that increasing one's intake of potassium can help reduce the risk of death by stroke or heart attack.[33] Since our cells need to maintain a ratio of twenty parts of potassium to one part of sodium, the increase of supplemental potassium and other essential elements such as magnesium and Vitamin C can greatly improve cellular activity. These three nutrients help to prevent the breakdown of arterial walls, the points where cholesterol accumulates to form plaque build-up.[34]

Myron H. Weinberger, director of the Hypertension Research Center at the Indiana University School of Medicine, has found evidence that sensitivity to sodium increases as people get older. Myron looked at a total of 650 people from 17 to 72 years of age, some with normal blood pressure and some with essential hypertension. To test sensitivity to sodium, subjects were given a large dose of salt water intravenously over a period of 4 hours, a process known as sodium loading. The next day, sodium intake was drastically reduced. The older hypertensives experienced greater increases in blood pressure after sodium loading, and greater decreases after depletion, than did the younger ones. In addition, sensitivity did not show up in subjects with normal blood pressure until after the age of fifty. The results also showed that hypertensives of any age will become more sensitive to sodium as they get older.[35]

Do you believe that when you have been perspiring a lot, you need to take some salt to restore your body's supply? Most of the time the answer is "no." When we sweat, our bodies take the opportunity to flush some of the excess salt that has been stored in our organs. The skin is our largest organ of elimination, though in most people this organ does not operate at its optimum. Sometimes the skin is called "the third kidney" because it takes over in the detoxification of the blood when our kidneys have more to do than they can handle. The skin eliminates, via perspiration, undesirable substances such as salt, uric acid, purines, and other toxic substances. Your body does not need salt to perspire and you needn't worry excessively about losing too much of it. A salt deficiency is a very rare malady.[36]

Rather, it is important to watch one's salt intake. In an optimum diet, salt should be kept to a minimum. If you desire the taste of salt, use it sparingly. Sea salt is the preferred salt to use; it contains a good assortment of trace minerals and actually has a better, though more subtle, flavor than processed salt.

Fiber

Get plenty of fiber in your diet. More people are aware of this need since the Surgeon General suggested in 1988 that Americans use oat bran instead of expensive drugs to lower cholesterol levels in the blood. All of a sudden, a commodity that was usually fed to pigs because of low demand became a premium item. Following their doctors' suggestions, people who would have never thought to venture in before began walking into health food stores.

Ironically, 1988 was also a drought year in the Midwest. This factor, together with low government subsidies to farmers who grew oats, managed to produce the smallest oat crop in 115 years. Needless to say, in the face of soaring demand, the American oat crop was soon depleted. Foreign sources were tapped. Ships with oat bran started arriving from Australia, Finland, Argentina, and other foreign ports. Of course, the price went up considerably. But, as usual, it was still much more economical to treat a cholesterol condition nutritionally than with the more expensive pharmaceutical drugs.

Some recent reports claim that oat bran only fills you up and does not really help reduce cholesterol, but I personally know people who have shown exceptional results when they added a significant amount of oat bran to their diets. The mechanism by which oat bran lowers cholesterol will be discussed in more detail when we look at the circulatory system.

The U.S. government has also been suggesting for some time that addition of high fiber foods to the diet is helpful in preventing colon cancer. Appendicitis, diverticulosis, hemorrhoids, constipation, allergies, and reabsorption of toxic waste products into the circulation (which encourages the development of degenerative diseases such as heart disease and arthritis) are also risks of a low-fiber diet.[37] Proper dietary levels of fiber are necessary to maintain a healthy digestive system and to keep bowel movements regular. The normal Western diet contains only ten to twenty grams of dietary fiber per day, while research points to the necessity of at least forty to sixty grams per day for optimum health.[38] It is interesting to note that the intestinal diseases that are so prevalent throughout the civilized world are almost unknown in rural Africa and many other societies where diets contain higher amounts of fiber.[39] In order to get twenty to thirty grams of fiber a day you would have to eat four ears of corn, three bowls of bran cereal, or twenty-five slices of white bread. There are many different kinds of fibers available in grains, vegetables, and fruits. But adding a supplement of extra fiber to your diet can only be beneficial.

Besides oat bran, bran from wheat, corn, and rice are all good sources of fiber. Fiber falls into several categories: cellulose, lignin, hemicellulose, pectin, and gums or mucilages. Cellulose and lignin are considered insoluble fibers because they pass through the digestive tract without breaking down. Insoluble fibers add roughage to our diet and tend to make bowel movements occur more regularly. Sources of insoluble fiber include fruits, vegetables, and wheat bran, which is about 99 percent insoluble. Pectin and gums (mucilages) are considered to be soluble fibers because they break down in the digestive tract. About one third of the fiber in fruits and vegetables is soluble and a few grains, such as oats, rice, and psyllium, have concentrated amounts of soluble fibers in their outer seed coatings, commonly known as the bran or husk. These soluble fibers are the ones that have been getting so much attention because of their effect on cholesterol levels. Hemicellulose is considered to have qualities of both insoluble and soluble fibers. An example of a hemicellulose is psyllium husks. Psyllium husks, the dried seed coat from the Plantago ovata plant of India, rank as one of the best soluble fibers available. They are gentle on the system, form soft bulky stools, and are more efficient in removing waste and toxins from the digestive system than any other form of fiber.[40]

Wheat bran, while widely used, has some less-than-favorable properties when taken in excess. It tends to be irritating to the lining of the digestive tract. In addition, there is some evidence that it tends to bind calcium and magnesium in such a way that the minerals become unavailable for absorption.[41] Using a combination of different fibers may be more beneficial than only using one type of fiber as a supplement.

Fiber supplements containing a variety of different plant fibers are available at your health food store. These products can be mixed with your food or sprinkled over cereal. You can even find natural candy bars that contain five or more types of fiber

Table 3.2   Fiber Content of Various Foods
(Average grams per 100 grams wet weight of food source)

Food	Total Plant Fiber	Insoluble Fiber	Soluble Fiber
Apple	2.0	1.1	0.9
Apple Fiber	40.0	30.0	10.0
Banana	1.8	1.0	0.8
Corn	3.2	1.8	1.8
Corn Flakes	12.2	5.0	7.2
Grape Nuts	13.0	7.4	5.6
Kidney Beans	10.2	5.5	4.7
Oat Bran	27.8	11.9	15.9
Oats, Rolled	13.9	6.2	7.7
Orange	2.0	1.4	0.6
Pinto Bean	10.5	6.0	4.5
Rice Bran	37.5	7.5	30.0
Sweet Potato	2.5	1.4	1.1
Wheat Bran	42.2	38.9	3.3
White Bean	7.7	4.0	3.7

Source: *Fiber Content of Various Foods*, TG Associates, Inc., Glenview, Illinois

for easy and tasty consumption. Refer to Table 3.2 for more about fiber.

Organically Grown

Americans are becoming increasingly aware of the possible "*cide*-effects" of eating fresh fruits and vegetables, as well as processed items derived from produce. Insecticides, fungicides, herbicides, acaricides, and rodenticides—these poisons protect our crops from insects, funguses, weeds, mites, and rodents. But in relying on them, are we taking the chance that we are poisoning ourselves as well? Are there natural alternatives for producing foods that are safer? These concerns are leading many people to turn to organically produced produce and products.

I've personally seen some of the hurtful effects of agricultural chemicals. I remember quite recently coming home to a very sick cat after a nearby field was sprayed with chemicals. The cat, which was in the house—not outside—drooled profusely for at least twelve hours and took days to recover. And many years ago, when I worked for a university entomology department mixing crop sprays, I spilled a drop of pesticide on my arm. Within minutes I was feeling dizzy and nauseous. Many of these products consist of very powerful chemicals; we ingest small amounts of them with most of the fresh produce we eat. I'm not trying to create hysteria, only trying to be informative about a subject that, until recently, has generally been ignored.

"Organic" is a term with a lot of different meanings, depending on whom you ask. The dictionary defines it as, "of, relating to, or derived from living organisms," and as, "of, relating to, or containing carbon compounds." The "organic" I am speaking about here is the definition of organic growing methods. Even when we narrow it down to this, however, we find differences in opinion between organic farmers and other farmers' groups. The California Organic Food Bill of 1979 defines organic produce as "agricultural commodities which are produced, stored, processed, and packaged without the use of synthetically compounded fertilizers, herbicides, fungicides, or pesticides for one year prior to the appearance of flower buds in the case of perennial crops and one year prior to seed planting in the case of annual crops." Other definitions prefer a two to three year period without the use of these compounds as residues often remain in the soil for several years. In the case of organic meat and dairy products, the animals are fed only organic grains and, in most cases, are not inoculated with growth hormones, vaccines, and other substances.

How important are chemical pesticides? Forty years ago, before they came into use, American farmers would lose 30 percent of their crops to insect pests. The amount lost to pest damage today is still 30 percent![42] So, with all the health hazards related to the extensive use of pesticides on the foods we eat, why not consider organic foods? After all, agricultural chemicals, in the form of chlorinated hydrocarbons, build up in high concentrations in our fatty tissues and remain for many years. Did you know that the average mother's milk in the United States has a concentration of pesticides exceeding the "acceptable daily intake" established for adults by the World Health Association?[43] In the late 1970s, the Environmental Protection Agency had found an average of two-and-a-half times the acceptable adult daily intake of DDE (DDT derivative in the body) in the milk of mothers they tested.[44] At the same time, a French study in 1974 showed pesticide residues in mother's milk to be less than half the norm in mothers eating a diet of 70 percent or more organically grown foods.[45]

Dioxin is another widely found, dangerous chemical residue accumulating in food products. It is most commonly known as a component of Agent Orange, the herbicide defoliant used in Vietnam that has harmed the health of so many of the veterans of that tragic war. It is also found in elevated levels in poultry, pork, beef, milk, eggs, and fish. A significant source of dioxin is in the wood preservative pentachlorophenol, used as sawdust for animal feed or around farms.

According to Barry Commoner, Ph.D., director of the Center for the Biology of Natural Systems at Queens College in New York City, current environmental levels of dioxin represent an increased cancer risk for at least 330 people out of every million.[46] Two hundred samples of mother's milk were evaluated for dioxin levels by Dr. Arnold Schecter, professor of preventive medicine at the State University of New York at Binghamton. He concluded that after one year of breast-feeding, North American babies are exceeding dioxin levels considered to be "maximum-lifetime" doses by most governments! Dr. Schecter and others are concerned by the indifference that the United States government has shown with regard to dioxin.[47]

Most of us are aware of the recent publicity about the growth regulator used on apples known as *Alar*. Alar (a trade name for the chemical *daminozide* produced by Uniroyal Chemical Company), when sprayed on apples, helps them ripen all at once, and preserves color and firmness so they can be marketed for many more months. It also helps the trees bloom every year instead of every other year.

On the CBS television show *60 Minutes*, where the use of this pesticide was again brought to the attention of the American public in February 1989, Alar was called "the most potent cancer-causing agent in our food supply!" Those who were most at risk were children whose diet consisted of more prepared apple products proportionate to their size than adults. Alar, when heated, generates a chemical known as UDMH, a known cancer-causing agent. Applesauce, baby food, pies, baked apples, and apple juice are all suspect due to the heating present in the processing of these products. The most astounding fact reported during the broadcast was that the EPA's acting administrator, Dr. Jack Moore, acknowledged that the EPA has known about the cancer risk for sixteen years.[48]

Even though most apple juice manufacturers issue statements saying that they no longer use Alar-treated apples in their products, when analyzed in the lab, the results of new tests were frightening. Two-thirds of thirty-two samples showed the presence of some degree of Alar. Alar and seven other pesticides have been researched by the Natural Resources Defense Council (NRDC). "It found the risk of developing cancer at 250 times what the EPA says is an acceptable level of cancer in our population," according to Janet Hathaway of NRDC. "One out of a million, they say, is acceptable." This is equivalent to one out of every 4,000 of our preschoolers having heightened exposure to the chance of developing cancer just from these eight pesticides.[49]

When the researchers at *Consumer Report Magazine* tested apple juice samples for three consecutive years, from 1987 to 1989, they were surprised to find almost no traces of Alar in the 1987 samples, while most of the 1988 and 1989 samples contained traces of the substance. They discovered they had used two different testing methods. The method used in 1987, known as the PAM II method, did not detect the presence of Alar below 0.5 parts per million. (Consumer Union's newer tests show that Alar is typically found in apples in levels of 0.2 to 0.5 parts per million.) Unfortunately, this error would also account for the fact that the National Food Processors Association could test more than 3,800 apples and find Alar detectable in only one sample.[50]

In 1970, pesticide regulation was transferred from the USDA to the EPA. At that time, some 320 pesticides were approved without extensive testing to document their safety. Since then, 66 of these pesticides have been classified as carcinogens by our government.[51] The scary thing is that the EPA doesn't know exactly what hazards many common pesticides may pose to humans. The EPA has only developed data on 192 of these older chemicals and today some 50,000 pesticide products in 600 chemical categories are being used.[52] This same EPA says pesticide residues pose the third-highest threat of environmentally induced cancer, behind first-ranking cigarettes and second-ranking radon.[53]

Even if the government improved its testing and regulation of the chemicals American farmers use on their crops, we would still obtain as much as 50 percent of our fruits and vegetables from abroad.[54] In many countries, pesticide use is not nearly as stringent as in our country. Benamil, a known carcinogen used on bananas in Latin American countries cannot be washed or peeled off. Over an 8-year period in the 1980s, 50 to 60 billion pounds of bananas came into the United States from South American countries. During this same period, the FDA sampled only two bananas for this dangerous compound![55] The point is that we certainly can't depend on government agencies to protect us from dangerous substances in our food supply.

Today, some supermarket chains are beginning to stock a variety of organic vegetables. In addition to the organic produce found in most natural food stores, there are many products on the shelves that contain organically grown ingredients. There are even a couple of organic baby food lines available. Sometimes, organic products cost a little bit more than similar, commercially grown items. But growing a quality product without chemicals is more labor-intensive and, therefore, more expensive. Producing an organic crop requires good management, including frequent monitoring for insects and, often, handpicking of the final product. Also, the quality of an organically grown product is better, in my opinion, than its potentially harmful counterpart. Though we may not always be able to find organically grown products, it makes sense to cut down our intake of harmful pesticides by obtaining these cleaner, more naturally grown commodities whenever we can. After all, who needs "cide-effects"!

Exercise

You can't maintain a healthy body without a regular pattern of physical exercise. Exercise provides activity and vigor to all the body's organs and supports the healthful integrity of their varied functions. It also improves the tone of muscle tissue and stimulates the processes of metabolism, digestion, absorption, and elimination. Cleansing of the system takes place as the body's toxins and waste products are eliminated through the pores when we work up a sweat. A regular exercise program will strengthen the heart, lungs, and blood vessels, which, in turn, will increase circulation and the flow of oxygen to the cells. The lymph system also benefits from this increased circulation.

Exercise can reduce the complications associated with diabetes and reduce the risk of heart disease. With regular activity, bone strength and muscle-tone are improved as well. Exercise not only stimulates the mind, it also helps to relieve stress and muscle tightness associated with stress. People who exercise claim that a regular workout makes them feel more relaxed and confident, less tired and irritable, as well as trimmer and stronger. In addition, a good exercise regime will help develop poise, grace, and body symmetry.

For some of you, yoga may be a consideration. Hatha yoga consists of stretching postures that provide a wonderful way to promote fitness, flexibility, and relaxation. Some other benefits of yoga include toning the body, calming the emotions, and steadying the mind. You may want to include some of these stretches with a more vigorous cardiovascular regime just to loosen up your muscles before and after your workout.

It is most beneficial to choose a program suited to one's own needs and abilities. Consult your doctor first. If you are just beginning an exercise regime, it is important to start out easy and gradually work your way up to a more rigorous workout. If you become impatient and push yourself too hard at first, you run the danger of straining yourself and actually slowing your progress. Be sure to wait at least one hour after eating (two is better) before engaging in exercise. Working out any sooner may impede digestion as well as cause discomfort.

Whether you start an exercise program to lose weight, to stay trim, or just to improve or maintain your health, some sort of aerobic exercise should be included in your regime. The term aerobic refers to the oxygen demand of the muscles. Tests have proven that just twelve to twenty minutes of proper aerobic exercising, three to six days a week, can greatly improve your health as well as reduce the fat content of your body. Some excellent examples of aerobic exercises are walking, running, jogging, running in place, cross-country skiing, jumping rope, outdoor or stationary cycling, rowing, dancing, swimming, roller skating, jumping jacks, and jumping on a mini-trampoline.

Proper aerobic exercising includes maintaining a certain rate of exercise determined by our pulse rates for a definite length of time. The rate at which we should exercise is approximately 80 percent of our maximum heart rate. A seasoned athlete may work at 85 percent of the maximum and someone with health problems—obesity or high blood pressure, for instance—will want to exercise at less than 75 percent of the maximum rate (under a doctor's supervision of course!). If you work out too strenuously by pushing your heart rate higher than recommended, you can actually do more harm and receive less benefit than by sticking to the optimum rate. (See Table 3.3 for recommended heart rates while exercising.) To determine your heart rate, find your pulse on your wrist near your thumb or on the side of your neck. Don't use your thumb to feel your pulse as it has a pulse of its own. Count how many pulse beats you have in a 6-second period and multiply this amount by 10 to get your heart rate. The accompanying chart is based on a resting heart rate of 72 for males and 80 for females. If you're over the age of 40 or have any heart problem, it's a good idea to have a stress electrocardiogram before starting an exercise program.

As mentioned earlier, to obtain optimum results from your aerobic workout, you must maintain this 80 percent heart rate for a definite period of time which is in many cases 12 minutes. If you work out for a shorter period of time you will gain very little benefit from your efforts. Also, two 6-minute periods do not add up in benefits to one 12-minute workout period. If you exercise for a longer period of time you will gain more benefit but not nearly as much as in the first 12 minutes. The main criterion of aerobic exercise is that it be steady and continuous.[57]

Table 3.3   Recommended Exercise Heart Rates

Age	Maximum Heart Rate	80% of Maximum (Recommended Training Rate)*
20	200	160
22	198	158
24	196	157
26	194	155
28	192	154
30	190	152
32	189	151
34	187	150
36	186	149
38	184	147
40	182	146
45	179	143
50	171	137
60	160	128
65+	150	120

Source: *Fit or Fat,* Covert Bailey, Houghton, Mifflin, Co.
*Note: If you have a heart condition, consult your doctor before undertaking an exercise program.

That means 12 minutes at the 80 percent heart rate. You should include a short warmup period before and a cool-down period after your aerobic workout as well. Three minutes of a similar exercise, only at a slower rate, is usually sufficient for each of these functions. Table 3.4 supplies minimum required times you should perform exercise for maximum effect.

Some individuals just love to exercise; but, for most of us, it takes a bit more effort to get motivated. Maintaining a successful exercise regime takes some will power, perseverance, and a sincere desire to improve one's physical condition. Make your

Table 3.4   Aerobic Exercise: Minimum Time Requirement

12 Minutes Minimum	15 Minutes Minimum	20 Minutes Minimum
Jumping Rope	Jogging	Walking
Jumping Jacks	Running	Swimming
Running-In-Place	Dancing	Bicycle (Outside)
	Mini-Trampoline	Stationary Bike
	Cross-County Skiing	Roller Skating
	Rowing	Ice Skating

Source: *Fit or Fat,* Covert Bailey, Houghton, Mifflin, Co.

exercise program self-motivating by doing what is enjoyable for you. An ideal exercise program may include many different types of physical activities. Choose the types of exercise that will interest you and be fun to do. Dancing, swimming, hiking, horseback riding, or a sport you really enjoy might be possibilities for you. Be sure to include some stretching exercises, or perhaps yoga postures, both before and after your regular regime. This will help prevent injury during exercise, as well as sore muscles after the workout.

A few more tips: Pick a time of day that is normally your own as well as an exercise you can do alone. Organized sports such as tennis or basketball tend to be more restrictive and time consuming. Watch television or listen to music to avoid boredom during exercise. Every once in a while supplement your routine with a different activity such as a team sport. Don't even think of missing your routine unless you are ill or injured. Just get out and do it! Work some flexibility into your program to accommodate business trips, rainy days, and other situations that may arise. And good luck with your fitness program.

Fasting and Cleansing

What we eat on an everyday basis and what we choose for our diet when we are experiencing a definite health problem are two different matters. When we are healthy there is room for a bit more leniency in our dietary habits. However, when we are stricken with a health problem, our body needs all the help it can get to fight off the condition. At such times, cleansing or fasting can be a helpful partner to the healing process.

Man may have learned from animals that fasting is an efficient means of treating disease. Animals, in most cases, stop eating when they are feeling ill. Digestion uses a great deal of the body's energy, and the less we eat when we are ill, the more energy is available to be used for the body's defenses. The actions of eliminatory organs like the kidneys, lungs, liver, and skin are greatly enhanced without the burden of digestion and the elimination of the waste products associated with digestion. Many clinical tests and scientific studies have been made, especially in Europe, concerning the therapeutic effects of fasting. Fasting is used in European and American clinics because of its rejuvenating and revitalizing effects and its ability to cleanse the body of accumulated wastes.

There are many different kinds of fasts, but the most common are water and juice fasting. Of these two, the latter is preferred because water fasting often leaves one in a weakened condition and in need of a recovery period afterward to regain one's normal strength. Contrary to this method, when we fast on fruit and vegetable juices, vegetable broth, and herb teas, we eliminate toxins and become revitalized at the same time, usually feeling stronger than when we started the fast. After three days our hunger typically becomes more manageable and fasting becomes easier. It is suggested we take long walks or engage in other exercise daily and use enemas to flush out toxins from our intestines while we are fasting. It is also recommended that the enemas be taken twice a day until three days after the fast is completed.

When fasting on fruit juice, after a few days you may find yourself getting a bit "spacy," (feeling like your head is in the clouds). The addition of carrot or beet juice will tend to ground you a bit, allowing for more clear thinking. Another general rule of cleansing is, "If it is green, it is cleansing." In other words, green-colored juices are high in chlorophyll, the substance that gives plants their characteristic green color. It is interesting to note that chlorophyll has almost the same chemical make-up as hemoglobin, the main constituent and oxygen carrier of our blood. There are a number of fine, "green" supplements, including liquid chlorophyll, green barley juice (available in a powder that you just add to juice or water), and fresh wheatgrass juice. All are high in minerals and very cleansing to the system. Be sensible about the length of time you fast and don't hesitate to consult your doctor if you are planning an extensive fasting program.

If fasting is not your style, other easier methods of internal cleansing are available as well. These other programs will usually take a little longer to cleanse the system but are generally a little more gentle and easy to incorporate into your everyday lifestyle. Yerba Prima Internal Cleansing Program is a simple way of cleansing the system while continuing to eat your normal diet. This program will be discussed in more detail in the discussion devoted to the colon.

Another simple technique that should be used with any cleansing program, and can be done on a daily basis whether cleansing or not, is called the dry-brush massage. The skin is our largest organ of elimination and, as mentioned before, is sometimes referred to as the "third kidney." Approximately one-third of all body impurities are eliminated by the skin. These waste products are passed through the pores of healthy skin via perspiration. (It is interesting to note that the chemical makeup of sweat is very similar to that of urine.) The liver, kidneys, and other organs of elimination tend to become overworked if these pores become clogged with dead cells, uric acid, and other impurities. Healthy skin actually assists in the breathing function by taking in oxygen and releasing carbon dioxide just like the lungs. There is also proof of the skin's ability to manufacture Vitamin D with the help of sunlight.[58] These functions are also inhibited by clogged pores.

By brushing your skin with a natural bristle brush, the dead cells and toxins that have accumulated and clogged the pores will be removed. This process will also stimulate the circulation under the skin and help rejuvenate the skin, resulting in better elimination and a softer, younger-looking complexion. Skin brushing also helps to flush and purify the lymph system. The lymph system serves as a storage area for cell waste and is essential for immune system functioning, our major defense against disease.

Be gentle when you begin a dry-brushing routine. It takes a while until your skin is "seasoned" to the point where a more stimulating brushing will be comfortable. Never use nylon or synthetic brushes as they can damage the skin. Also don't brush the face or any part of the skin that is overly sensitive or irritated. Using a natural bristle brush or a loofah mitt, both available at your natural foods store, brush your whole body in circular motions as hard as is comfortable. Some people will have more sensitive skin and need a softer stroke and different parts of the body will require different pressure. Brush until the skin is rosy and warm, and then take a shower to wash off the loosened cells and toxins. Be sure to brush when the skin is dry as it may cause sagging if the skin is wet.[59] This regime can be repeated once or twice a day.

Sluggish metabolism and inefficient elimination cause the body to retain and accumulate toxic wastes in the cells, which, in turn, interfere with their nourishment. Cells and tissues that do not receive proper nutrition become prone to disease. Many people like to do some sort of cleansing process at intervals during the year. This practice helps maintain the body's defense systems at their optimum levels and, thus, assists in the prevention of health problems.

Enjoying Your Food

This information has been presented to give you some guidelines to improve your diet, but I firmly believe that being too rigid in our dietary goals can lead to stress, which is in itself detrimental to our health. Some personalities may function perfectly well with a strict regime, but for most people, the first steps are to learn what foods are unhealthy, to discover what healthy alternatives exist, and then slowly to make the transition to a better diet. Usually, as we start to read labels and seek out better alternatives to the junk foods we have been in the habit of eating, we start to discover that there are a great many delicious products in the natural foods category. These were foods that we once thought would contain only boring and distasteful possibilities.

Both the body and the psyche need an adjustment period when a dietary change is taking place. If you change your diet too abruptly, you will probably experience some discomfort and may very well become discouraged. Be gentle with yourself. Don't try to force a change. Instead, enjoy the discovery of new horizons in cuisine. Make a firm resolution to improve your diet and health and look for ways to comfortably achieve these goals.

I encourage any of you not in the habit of visiting natural foods stores to go into one and browse a little. You may be pleasantly surprised. Now make sure it is a natural foods store containing a full range of products and not just a health food store you check out. The difference is the latter is predominantly a "supplement shop" and though many health food stores are fine establishments, they may not provide you with a real understanding of the variety of interesting foods that are now available. If you see something you like, ask someone who works there about it. The personnel in natural foods stores are generally willing to help you because they know that many people need to be educated about their products.

There are also some good reference books available that can help you learn about the variety of natural foods available. *Shopper's Guide to Natural Foods* from the editors of the *EastWest Journal* provides some excellent purchasing and preparation information for consumers. *Natural Foods and Good Cooking* by Kathy Cituk and John Finnegan offers a good basis to understand different natural food products along with a host of fine recipes. Another informative text for learning to cook with natural foods is *Natural Foods Cookbook* by Mary Estella. These and other fine books available at your local natural foods store can speed up your learning of the subtleties associated with the variety of nutritious foods available to you.

So, educating ourselves to upgrade our diets, reading labels to know what we are eating, and enjoying the foods we eat are all steps to a better diet. These practices, together with using common sense and moderation in our indulgence of "poor" foods, is the best regime I can recommend to help you achieve a healthier lifestyle.

Part Two

Healing Partners: Natural Medicines

We've examined the elaborate network of natural defenses inherent within the body. Whether we suffer from ill health caused by accident, environmental conditions, or our own bad habits, the systems of the body go to work to restore and maintain a healthful condition. Even without any conscious help from us, a somewhat healthy body is equipped to combat and correct most health problems. We do, however, have at our disposal an arsenal of quality natural healing products and techniques to act as allies in our body's defense program. In this section, I hope to introduce you to many of these healing aids.

4

The Digestive System

The digestive system has three primary functions: digestion, absorption, and elimination. Digestion is the process that takes large food molecules and breaks them down into simpler nutrient molecules so they can easily be used by the cells of the body. Absorption is the process by which these nutrient molecules are transferred across the lining that separates the digestive tract from the bloodstream. Once in the bloodstream, these nutrients can be delivered to the cells. The final process, elimination, removes from the body the leftover wastes of ingested foods.

The digestive tract, also called the alimentary tract or the gastrointestinal tract, extends from the mouth to the anus and is made up of numerous organs. Food placed in the mouth is broken down into smaller pieces by the teeth and mixed with the digestive enzymes of the saliva by the tongue. The tongue then pushes the mixture back into the throat where it initiates a muscular wave propelling it through the pharynx and esophagus to the stomach.

The stomach, the most widened portion of the digestive tract, has three functions: to store food, to mix it with digestive secretions to form a partly digested mass called chyme, and to empty the chyme into the small intestine slowly enough to permit proper digestion and absorption.

The next leg of our digestive journey takes us to the organ called the small intestine, which, contrary to its name, measures about eighteen feet in length. The digestive juices of the liver and pancreas are secreted into the upper portion of this enormously long organ. The intestine itself contains numerous intestinal glands that secrete a major portion of the digestive enzymes into the intestinal contents. The primary functions of the small intestine are chemical digestion and absorption of nutrients.

The intestinal contents then move on to the large intestine or colon where no digestive juices are secreted. The main function of the colon is to absorb some nutrients and excess water, as digestive juices are made up of approximately 95 percent water. The remaining solid waste or feces is moved on to the rectum where it is eliminated through the anal canal.

Keeping this system working efficiently is essential to all the cells and tissues of the body. It is here that food is made available to the rest of the body and many toxic substances are removed before they are a threat to the health of other tissues and organs. In this chapter, I will discuss some common ailments that affect the digestive organs and some products available that may initiate some relief for these problems.

Mouth Sores

Sores in or on the mouth can be especially annoying and painful, kindling a kind of misery way out of proportion to their tiny size. These pesty sores often resist the treatment modern medicine has developed to reduce their severity. Usually called cold sores, canker sores, or fever blisters, they occur on the edge of the tongue, the gums, and the lips. These sores are associated with the herpes virus and, although a person may not suffer from them for a good portion of his or her life, once he or she gets a cold sore it is likely to recur. These infections often occur when the body is under stress from either mental or emotional influences or from a physical illness. Some people may get fever blisters from too much sun or an allergic reaction. Others can get mouth sores from an over-acid condition caused by an excess of sugar in the diet.

Some Natural Products Used to Treat Mouth Sores:

☐ **Hyland's Calendula Off. Tincture:** A homeopathic preparation used on mouth sores to aid in healing. Apply topically.
☐ **Bach Rescue Remedy:** A flower remedy used for coping with the stress that often contributes to mouth sore formation.
☐ **Yerba Prima Adaptoplex:** An herbal formulation used for coping with the stress that often contributes to mouth sore formation.

☐ **Zand Lysine Herbal:** Lysine supplementation has been shown to retard mouth sore formation.

☐ **Nature's Way Primadophilus:** Studies show acidophilus supplements help relieve mouth sore problems.

☐ **Yerba Prima Fiberdophilus:** Studies show acidophilus supplements help relieve mouth sore problems.

☐ **Energy Medicine Fever Blister or Canker Sore:** A homeopathic formulation used for the relief of mouth sore symptoms.

I've found a homeopathic solution of calendula (made from the marigold flower) often helps with the pain of canker sores and may speed their disappearance. Hyland's Calendula Off. Tincture solution is a high-quality preparation produced by Standard Homeopathic. A mixture of one part Calendula to three parts water swished around in the mouth hourly has helped me in the past when I suffered from this problem. I once had a friend who needed to have gum grafts performed in his mouth. He tried this treatment and he reported the oral surgeon could not believe how quickly his mouth had healed.

Since stress seems to irritate canker sores, some benefit might result from taking Bach Rescue Remedy or Adaptoplex (discussed in Chapter 6), both of which are designed to help ease any mental anxiety resulting from the pain or other influences. By the way, if you are suffering from a sore in the mouth, it pays to eat soft food because these little ulcers take longer to heal when irritated by rough foods.

The amino acid L-lysine has become a popular supplement due to medical reports showing its effectiveness in treating the herpes simplex virus. Back in 1974, a research group found that when herpes invaded a cell, it changed the metabolism resulting in a correspondence between the amino acids arginine and lysine. It was postulated that, since a high arginine-to-lysine ratio was found with herpes, the opposite ratio might control the problem. Studies revealed that a high level of lysine in the blood showed a decrease in the recurrence rate of herpes outbreaks; low levels of lysine in the blood increased this recurrence rate.[1]

In a more recent study at the Indiana University School of Medicine, 1000 mg. of lysine were administered to herpes sufferers on a daily basis. A full 84 percent of the subjects reported that the lysine had prevented recurrence or decreased the frequency of infection. Ninety-two percent reported a reduction in the pain suffered from the herpes outbreaks and, in most cases, the healing period was reduced by a number of days.[2]

An excellent dietary supplement known as Zand Lysine Herbal is produced by Zand Herbal Formulas. Formulated by Dr. Janet Zand, this formula combines lysine with a selected blend of herbs and nutrients to provide wonderful dietary additions to those who suffer from herpes-type infections, including Epstein Barr virus.

Another study performed back in the 1950s at Peter Bent Brigham Hospital in Boston revealed an additional supplement effective in relieving the symptoms of mouth sores. Dr. Don J. Weeks was treating several patients suffering from diarrhea with tablets containing *Lactobacillus acidophilus* and *Lactobacillus bulgaricus*, beneficial bacteria used to culture yogurt and other sour milk products. Two of his patients were also suffering from severe canker sores and, after taking the tablets, the sores showed dramatic improvement. Dr. Weeks decided to try the lactobacillus treatment on other canker sore sufferers. He published the results of his two studies in medical journals in 1958 and 1963.

One test of Dr. Weeks involved 174 patients from the ages of 2 to 66, all with painful blisters or sores in or about the mouth. In each case, the subject was advised to take four L. acidophilus-bulgaricus tablets 4 times a day with some milk. Among the 64 patients treated for fever blisters on the lip, 37 obtained complete relief and another 24 showed great improvement. This translates to 95 percent of the subjects showing favorable results. Not only did the supplement soothe and speed the healing of the blisters, but in some cases it actually prevented the recurrence of new sores. In the case of the other 97 patients with canker sores in the mouth, 80 percent experienced a favorable result. Dr. Weeks also stated that when used in the early stages of canker sore development, acidophilus will actually abort imminent lesions.[3]

Research shows that if you are troubled by frequent outbursts of fever blisters, cold or canker sores, a supplement of eight to twelve acidophilus capsules per day may benefit you. Live yogurts don't contain enough acidophilus to give you these potencies and most yogurts you buy commercially, if not pasturized to kill all beneficial bacteria, lack the acidophilus strain.

There are several good acidophilus supplements on the market, but two I prefer are Nature's Way Primadophilus and Yerba Prima Fiberdophilus. The Nature's Way product is a high-potency concentrate containing over 10 billion microorganisms per gram. Containing no dairy products, soy, corn, wheat, or yeast, it is hypoallergenic. In addition it comes in a capsule that is "enterosoluble." This, according to Nature's Way, means the active microorganisms are not released until they reach the intestines, thereby solving the problem that some capsules break down in the stomach where many of the microorganisms are destroyed, never to reach the intestines where they are needed. The capsule can only be broken down in the intestines because of the difference in pH levels in this section of the digestive tract.

Another fine acidophilus supplement is Yerba Prima Fiberdophilus. This product, which combines lactobacillus acidophilus with fiber, not only provides the pH level preferred by the acidophilus (5.0-7.0), but also provides barley malt extract, a nutrient that speeds acidophilus growth in the colon. The result is a product that enriches the intestinal flora while neutralizing and removing toxic waste products in the colon.[4]

If you are interested in trying a homeopathic medication for canker sores or fever blisters, there is a fine formula available. Dolisos America Inc. manufacturers a product specifically for mouth sores. Energy Medicine Fever Blister or Canker Sore is their formulation of six homeopathic preparations that stimulate the body defenses to help with these conditions.

If acidity in the body is the cause of recurrent canker and other mouth-sore problems, another product may be of help. Common baking soda, found in most households, has been known to bring down the body's pH level to a place where the herpes simplex virus does not thrive. For years I was personally plagued by extremely painful canker sores. I observed that when I ate too much sugar, a canker sore would develop. I became so sensitive that I could not even eat fruit, drink fruit juice, or tolerate any sweeteners at all.

At the suggestion of a friend who referred me to a book by Angela Kilmartin entitled *Cystitis, The Complete Self-Help Guide*, I began to take one-quarter teaspoon of baking soda every day. I took the baking soda early in the morning as I found that, taken immediately before eating, it interfered with my digestion. After several weeks, I found I could eat sweets again and not be infected as easily by canker sores. I still find if I really overindulge in sweets, I am prone to canker sores. But baking soda has helped to make me less sensitive. Doctors have noted that one teaspoonful an hour for three or four hours is an acceptable dose and does not result in any side effects.[5] However, anyone with blood pressure problems or heart conditions should discuss this technique with their family physician before trying it.

By the way, adding carbon dioxide to the blood will lower the pH level of the blood. Because exercising causes deeper and more rapid breathing and accelerated breathing removes carbon dioxide from the blood, simply exercising more might lower the acidity level of the blood!

Other studies have shown that large doses of B vitamins, especially B-12 and folic acid, may build your resistance to mouth sores. Carlton Fredericks, Ph.D. notes, "Persistent and very severe cold sores in a seven-year-old child who was taking numerous vitamin-mineral supplements, and which responded to no type of medical treatment, disappeared when 250 micrograms of Vitamin B-12 were added to the treatment."[6] A deficiency of iron has also been shown to increase susceptibility to mouth sores.

So, if you suffer from painful and irritating recurrences of canker sores, cold sores, or fever blisters, you might want to experiment with some of these supplements. Perhaps a deficiency in your system can be relieved with a supplementation of lysine, acidophilus, or B vitamins. Or maybe adjusting your blood pH with a little baking soda is all that is necessary. I combine several of these strategies when the first signs of these conditions begin to occur.

Indigestion and Nausea

We all have suffered from a stomach ache or other stomach discomfort at some time or another. The usual cause of stomach trouble is diet and eating habits. If we don't chew our foods thoroughly, the stomach has to work harder to break down our food substances. As I have already mentioned, food needs to be chewed well and mixed with saliva until it is in a semi-liquid state before it is swallowed. The saliva is the liquid that starts the process of carbohydrate digestion and if we do not chew thoroughly enough, or if we dilute our food with an excess of liquids, this step in the process is neglected. If this first step in the breakdown of carbohydrates does not occur adequately, food substances may ferment in the stomach and cause gas and discomfort.

Live enzymes are needed to digest our foods and even to allow vitamins, minerals, and hormones to do their work. Enzymes in the food we eat are meant to contribute to our digestive effort. Raw foods are full of live enzymes, but when we heat our food by cooking or processing, the enzymes are inactivated. Whenever we allow our foods to boil at 212°F, all enzymes are completely destroyed.[7] The stomach is designed with an upper "cardiac" region where enzymes are not secreted. This portion of the stomach is designed to hold the food for a period of time while the enzymes in the food and the saliva start to break it down. This can happen effectively if we are eating mostly raw foods. Because so much of our society's diet consists of cooked or processed foods, this often does not occur, however. As a result, our pancreas and other enzyme-secreting organs become overworked and eventually stressed.[8]

In experiments at Michael Reese Hospital in Chicago, it was found that young adults between the ages of 21 to 31 years of age had 30 times more amylase, a salivary enzyme that breaks down starch, than older adults between the ages of 69 to 100. This and other research suggests that our enzyme reserve becomes depleted as we become older.[9] There is also a relationship between chronic diseases and the levels of enzymes available in the body. In a Japanese study involving 111 tuberculosis patients, 82 percent of them had lower enzyme contents than normal individuals. It is a documented fact that during episodes of chronic disease (periods marked by long duration or frequent recurrence), we find a lower enzyme content in blood, urine, feces, and tissues.[10] Dr. Edward Howell, a pioneer in enzyme research, maintains that ill health, and ultimately our death, occurs when our enzyme production capabilities finally become exhausted.[11] Because of the importance of enzymes to our health, it would not hurt to consider adding more fresh foods, and possibly some enzyme supplements, to our diets.

Digestion in the stomach occurs by two means, mechanical and chemical. Wave-like contractions churn the food while digestive enzymes break down the food molecules into smaller, more assimilative units. When we ingest the wrong combinations of foods or eat foods such as chemical food additives that are not easily digestible, they may coat the lining of the stomach and inhibit the secretion of digestive juices. When this takes place, an over-acid condition may develop. Since the stomach is also a storage unit for the chyme while it is slowly released to the intestines, this acidic mass may remain in the stomach for a prolonged period, causing further irritation. This results in one or more uncomfortable conditions including gas, heartburn, bloating, and indigestion.

The stomach needs to relax to digest foods correctly. Stress and eating on the run often lead to indigestion. Stop your busy pace of life when you sit down to eat. If need be, find a quiet, private place to enjoy your food and just stop and close your eyes for a few minutes to slow everything down before you begin your meal. By taking the time to eat slower, you will not only taste and enjoy your food more, but you will tend to feel better after you have finished.

Other causes of stomach problems include too many greasy, spicy, or refined foods, alcohol, vinegar, and caffeine. Eating too much at one time can also put pressure on the stomach and dilute the digestive juices so they work less efficiently. Be sure to watch your intake so as not to "stuff" yourself. Eating slower will also help you to stop before you are too full.

Sometimes the combinations of foods we eat can also work against the digestion process. Of the several different theories concerning food-combining, perhaps the best known is not to mix fruits with vegetables. Unfortunately, I could never find any practical evidence to substantiate this theory. To me the most legitimate food-combining system is the one favored by Dr. Randolph Stone, the founder of polarity therapy. This system points out the two different digestion processes taking place in the stomach, the first being protein digestion (which needs an acidic medium to accomplish its task), and the second being carbohydrate digestion (which needs an alkaline pH to function effectively). Eating a heavy protein with a starch or sugar (i.e., a hamburger on a bun) at the same meal creates a situation where the stomach acid works on the protein and the carbohydrate has to wait. If the stomach does not empty out quickly, the carbohydrate can start to ferment and form an excess of organic acids that leads to heartburn. The next thing most people tend to do is take an antacid, neutralizing the stomach acid and retarding the process of protein digestion.

Dr. Stone suggests the best combinations are alkaline fruits (sweet fruits and juices such as figs, dates, raisins, prunes, and/ or prune juice) with carbohydrate foods (breads, cakes, cereals, grains, and/or potatoes). He also recommends mixing acidic fruits (grapefruit, oranges, orange juice, and/or lemonade) with foods high in protein (eggs, meat, cheese, and/or tofu). Most vegetables, he says, can be mixed with anything. From my experience, these simple rules not only make sense, but work. You also may find that your digestion improves when you follow these guidelines. Food combining has its shortcomings, however, as many foods contain both proteins and carbohydrates and it can be a little excessive to try to practice it religiously. But when you have a definite digestive problem it may help to pay attention to your combinations, at least until the problem subsides.

Some Natural Products Used for Indigestion and Related Disturbances:

☐ **Yerba Prima Chamomile:** An herb with properties that are calming and soothing to the digestive system.

☐ **Zand Digest Herbal Formula:** An herbal formula that relieves gastric distress and that bloated feeling after overeating.

☐ **Power Herbs Digest-Ease:** An herbal formula that relieves gastric distress, bloating, and pains associated with gas.

☐ **Floradix Herbal Bitters:** Bitter herbs assist in the digestion of heavy and fatty foods.

☐ **Yerba Prima Aloe Vera plus Herbs:** An herbal juice that is soothing and healing to the digestive tract.

☐ **Energy Medicine Nausea (Vomiting):** A homeopathic formulation used for relief of the symptoms of nausea and
vomiting.

☐ **Rainbow Light All-Zyme:** An herbal supplement that contains all four food enzyme groups and acts as an enzyme
replacement and digestive aid.

When indigestion does occur, there are non-prescription
products available that may offer some relief. There are plenty
of antacids on the market, but most of these contain aluminum
compounds, which have been shown to deplete calcium in the
body when used continually. Calcium depletion can result in
thinning of bones and bone pain. There are also other health
problems that have been associated with the ingestion of aluminum products. Suffice it to say, it is best to steer clear of products containing aluminum compounds.

Some effective natural alternatives are available and you
might consider experimenting with them the next time you are
suffering from heartburn, indigestion, or a stomach upset.
Yerba Prima Chamomile is a standardized herbal product in
tablet form, containing a concentration of the chamomile herb.
This herb is known for its calming and soothing qualities on the
digestive system as well as its role as a bitter. Bitters are traditionally used in Europe for stomach problems. They are also
calming to the mind so they can make you a little sleepy.

Zand Herbal Formulas produces an excellent product as a digestive aid that promotes digestion naturally, without the use of
animal products or enzymes. This product is Zand Digest
Herbal Formula. The active ingredient, peppermint spirit, is
combined with a carefully selected combination of fine bitter
herbs. Current research indicates that peppermint relieves gastric distress by causing the stomach to empty earlier than usual.[12]
The bitter herbs goldenseal and gentian also have an extensive
history of use to invigorate digestion. Their combination is capable of relieving the bloated feeling associated with overeating.

Another digestive product is Power Herbs Digest-Ease, produced by Nature's Herbs. This preparation combines many excellent botanicals as well as several standardized quantities of
digestive enzymes from plant origins. Enzymes include papain

and prolase from papaya for protein digestion, bromelain from pineapple for protein digestion, diastase from barley malt for carbohydrate digestion, and amylase from *Aspergillus oryzae* for digesting starches. In addition, other herbs such as peppermint, chamomile, and slippery elm are included for their soothing qualities. This product works with your body to provide relief of stomach and intestinal distress, bloating, distention, fullness, pressure, pain, or cramps (gas) that occur after eating. It also enhances the normal digestion processes.[13] From my experience, this product usually provides me with very fast relief when I have an upset stomach.

Floradix Herbal Bitters is an exceptional West German supplement, which aids the digestive process. This product contains artichoke and nine selected herbs to assist appetite and digestion when taken at mealtime. Bitter herbs have been used since the time of the ancient Greeks to support digestion, liver, and gall bladder functioning. According to Mark Blumenthal, herbal researcher and writer, "Many bitter herbs have the physiological effect of activating digestive fluids in the salivary glands and stomach."[14] This liquid extract formula promotes necessary bile flow, which assists in the digestion of fatty and heavy foods. This, in turn, relieves congestion and flatulence and helps avoid that full feeling after rich meals. Floradix Herbal Bitters does not contain any alcohol as do many of the bitter formulations on the market.

Aloe vera is another herb that is capable of bringing some relief from stomach discomfort. It is very soothing and healing to mucous membranes, and the entire digestive system can benefit from this supplement. Yerba Prima produces another excellent product: Yerba Prima Aloe Vera plus Herbs. Though some people like the taste of aloe, some may have tasted bitter aloe juice and prefer it mixed with fruit juice. There are flavored aloes available, but many have questionable ingredients. Yerba's aloe vera product is made from the inner gel of the aloe leaf and the bitterness associated with aloe is usually due to the presence of the bitter outer rind. The herbs added to this aloe product—peppermint, parsley, and chapparal—are known for their cleansing, purifying, and soothing qualities, and enhance the flavor of the juice as well. If your purpose is to soothe an acidic stomach, you don't want to mix too much fruit juice with your aloe as the fruit juice is quite acidic in itself.

Another unpleasant condition associated with stomach upset is nausea, which in more severe cases may lead to the discharging of the stomach contents, which is commonly known as vomiting. Vomiting is a mechanism that nature has provided to help us eliminate toxic substances from the body before they cause us additional harm. A homeopathic alternative for the possible relief of nausea or vomiting is produced by the Dolisos America Inc. This formulation of five homeopathic medications is called Energy Medicine Nausea (Vomiting). Each of the five components help the body's defenses to remedy the uncomfortable feelings associated with these conditions. Motion sickness, another ailment involving nausea, will be addressed in Chapter 6.

If you want to assist the digestive process, Rainbow Light Nutritional Systems provides an excellent enzyme supplement and digestive aid to add to your diet. Rainbow Light All-Zyme blends highly active potencies of all four food enzyme groups into a balanced formula designed for enzyme replacement, as well as for the digestion of well-balanced meals. These four enzyme categories consist of:

1. Lipase, which serves to break down fats;
2. Protease, which serves to break down proteins;
3. Cellulase, which serves to break down cellulose; and
4. Amylase, which serves to break down starch.

Each of these enzyme categories include several different enzymes. All-Zyme is ideal for those who eat meals consisting of a variety of foods containing proteins, carbohydrates, and fats.[15] Enzymes are also used up faster during certain illnesses, during extremely hot or cold weather, and during strenuous exercise.[16] Also keep in mind that enzymes taken are added to what is known as the enzyme pool of your body and are therefore never wasted.[17] This product approaches a solution to the lack of live enzymes in most of our diets. It is designed to be taken with your meals and is guaranteed by Rainbow Light to give you satisfactory results within thirty days.

The best thing you can do for your stomach is to learn to improve your eating habits. Don't eat too much at one sitting and chew your food well. Don't drink so much liquid during the meal that the digestive enzymes become overly diluted. Find a quiet place to eat where you can slow down and enjoy your food. Also, try to eat simpler, less-processed foods, especially if you have a persistent problem, so your stomach can do its work to regain its function as an efficient organ of digestion.

Stomach Ulcers

Statistically, one in every ten persons is likely to suffer from peptic ulcers and see their physician for treatment, but many more will be lightly affected and never consult a doctor. This condition is increasing in incidence at a fairly rapid rate.[18] Most people are aware that stomach ulcers are the result of the over-action of digestive acids on the lining of the stomach. However, an ulcerous condition is not always due to excess acid secretion. *Guyton's Basic Human Physiology* describes the cause of stomach ulcers: "Gastric ulcers occur in patients who have normal or high secretion of HCl (hydrochloric acid) . . . ulceration in the stomach almost certainly results from reduced resistance of the stomach mucosa to digestion rather than excess secretion of gastric juice." Guyton also claims that aspirin and alcohol reduce mucosal resistance. Of course, if the mucosal lining of the stomach is in a weakened state, excess acid will only do more harm. Stress will cause increased HCl secretions in the stomach and is probably the most common suspect in the event of stomach ulcers. Other substances that can cause an increased acid condition are spicy foods, cigarette smoke, and certain medications including cortisone, reserpine, aspirin, and prednisone.

If you suffer from an ailment as serious as an ulcer, hopefully you are already in the care of a doctor. He or she has probably instructed you to reduce the stress in your life, drink lots of water, exercise (which also helps to relieve stress), and perhaps get lots of sun. He or she may also have you on medication. You should follow your doctor's instructions, of course, but at the same time, we do have a few suggestions to make.

Some Natural Products Used for Stomach Ulcers:

☐ **Yerba Prima Adaptoplex:** An herbal formula that helps reduce the stress that can lead to stomach ulcers.

☐ **Hyland's Calms:** A homeopathic formulation used to relieve simple nervous tension that can lead to stomach ulcers.

☐ **Yerba Prima Aloe Vera plus Herbs:** An herbal juice that is soothing and healing to the digestive tract.

There are two Yerba Prima supplements that I would add to my diet if I had a stomach ulcer. The first is a product commonly taken for stress, Yerba Prima Adaptoplex. Adaptoplex works to relax tension induced by stress while helping to improve energy. This product will be discussed in detail under the subject of stress.

At a time of rapid growth at a natural foods company for which I worked, I was experiencing a lot of stress. In fact, I felt so tense that I actually started to become ill. Of the other two people in the office, one had already been sick from simple burn-out and the other looked so worn out that I hoped I didn't look as bad. I tried a couple of Adaptoplex and within a short time felt the "nervous edge" begin to melt away. Since that time, I have found that this product has helped balance the effects of stress on many occasions. If I expect a stress-filled day ahead, I will often take two tablets before work just for insurance. If stress is causing your ulcerous condition, you might consider asking your physician if you can include this product in your supplement program.

Another product already mentioned under less serious stomach disorders for its soothing, healing properties, is Yerba Prima Aloe Vera plus Herbs. Research has been done treating ulcer patients with aloe vera juice. One such research project involved twelve patients diagnosed with serious stomach ulcers accompanied with duodenal cap lesions. All these patients had recovered completely after taking generous dosages of aloe vera on a daily basis. After recovery, small dosages were taken daily to prevent recurrence of the problem. Usually such unmistakable lesions are accompanied with future occurrences of distress once or twice a year after being relieved by any form of standard medical treatment. No such episodes were experienced in any of these patients, even after a period of eighteen months at which time this research was concluded.[19]

I know that if I suffered from a peptic ulcer, I wouldn't hesitate to take at least eight ounces of aloe vera juice several times each day until the condition corrected itself, even if I were under medication for this problem. I would also take small doses on a daily basis, before bed, for a year or two after the condition disappeared, just to help prevent additional problems from occurring.

Another product that can help with stress-related symptoms, which will also be looked at in more detail when we discuss stress later in the book, is Hyland's Calms. This homeopathic combination, consisting of four different remedies for stress-type symptoms, can also offer a safe means of relieving the stress associated with ulcerous conditions.

In another test by a Dr. Frommer in Sydney, Australia, the beneficial effects of a zinc supplement on ulcer patients was studied. Of eighteen patients, ten were given ninety milligrams of zinc sulfate three times a day while the other eight were given placebos. Neither doctors nor patients knew who was receiving the zinc. The results indicated that the patients taking the zinc supplement had three times the healing rate than that of the placebo takers. No side effects from the zinc sulfate were observed.[20]

So if you have or suspect you might have an ulcer, be sure to consult a physician, as this can be a very serious condition. At the same time, you might consider a zinc supplement, Aloe Vera plus Herbs, and Adaptoplex as additions to your diet.

Constipation and Diarrhea

The colon or large intestine is an organ of digestion measuring approximately five feet in length. Its main functions are the absorption, storage, and transportation of fecal material. It is the home of over fifty different microorganisms such as bacteria, yeast, fungi, and possibly, in cases of infection, amoebae. If the colon bacteria are normal, they produce Vitamins B-1, B-2, B-12, and K. All, with the possible exception of B-12, are absorbed through the colon wall for use by the body. A good population of beneficial bacteria also inhibits the growth of toxin-producing microorganisms, reduces cholesterol content of the blood, and by producing natural antibiotics, inhibits many pathogenic organisms.[21] Maintaining a healthy bacterial population in the colon is important in achieving optimum health. In a healthy condition, over 80 percent of the material reaching the large intestine is reabsorbed.[22](See figure on page 81.)

Unfortunately, a healthy colon is a rare occurrence in modern society. Poor-quality foods of low fiber content along with poor exercise and eating habits, some of which were already mentioned, result in a slower movement of fecal material through the colon. Some of this material is of mucoid nature, which tends to be of a sticky, gluey consistency. This mucoid matter deposits itself on the wall of the intestine and over a period of many years, a thick residue of tough, rubbery black substance may build up. This coating interferes with the colon's normal absorption function and provides a welcome environment for harmful microorganisms, parasites, and other detrimental intruders. Certain harmful bacteria in the *clostridium family* have the ability to take substances such as bile acids, cholesterol, and fatty acids and convert them into toxic substances, including cancer-producing agents.

Old feces may build up in pockets of the colon or coat the entire lining of this organ and the small intestine as well (see illustration). These residues are not eliminated from the body with normal bowel movements, but require special cleansing techniques to dissolve them.[23] Therefore, there is a better than average chance that your colon is packed with a lifetime's accumulation of old, hardened fecal material.

Accumulation of old feces in the colon can also stretch the organ out of shape. At birth, we have a relatively uniform series of pouch-like sacs that make up the colon. X-ray studies have clearly shown that fecal deposits deform the shape and position of the intestine, leading to a number of problems, the most obvious being constrictions that obstruct the passage of fecal material. Even with a good cleansing program, it may take years utilizing good eating habits to restore the colon to its normal shape. Nevertheless, removing the abdominal pressure by cleansing the colon is an essential step in relieving any discomfort and restoring the normal functioning and structure to this organ.

Some authorities claim that virtually every disease begins with a toxic colon. This premise would be difficult to verify. Suffice it to say that if the colon is not able to produce or absorb vital nutrients (due to absence of beneficial bacteria or a coating

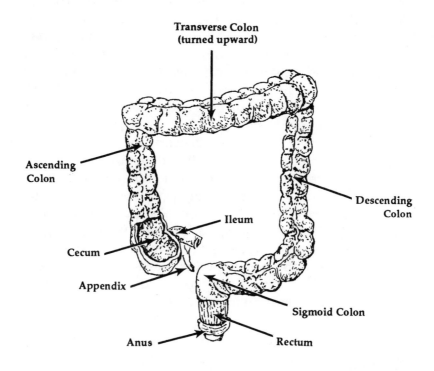

Normal Colon

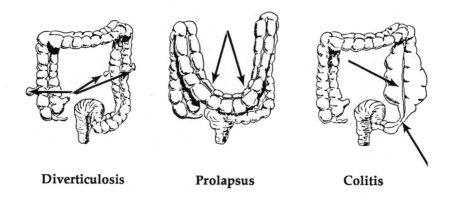

Diverticulosis　　　**Prolapsus**　　　**Colitis**

COLON DYSFUNCTIONS

of mucoid matter), we are looking at an unhealthy condition. Also, if the time required for the fecal matter to move through the colon (known as the transit time) is slower than optimum, the fecal matter will putrefy and release additional toxins to be absorbed by the body. The body is weakened by the presence of toxins, parasites, etc. due to this unhealthy condition in the colon, so it stands to reason that the body's healing strength could very well be compromised.

In addition, when the bowel is overworked or not functioning properly, the body will try to find other avenues of elimination. Some symptoms of these elimination attempts due to a toxic colon condition include: skin problems, frequent congestion, colds, virus, headaches, aches and pains, lowered resistance to infections, low energy, bad breath, foul-smelling stool, flatulence, allergies, premenstrual syndrome, vaginal infections, and bowel problems.[24] While gastrointestinal cleansing will not cure disease, it certainly could aid the body defenses in overcoming disease if our elimination system is operating optimally.

Some Natural Products Used for Colon Problems:

☐ **Nature's Way Cascara Sagrada:** An herb with laxative and toning properties.

☐ **Nature's Herbs Cascara Sagrada:** An herb with laxative and toning properties.

☐ **Energy Medicine Constipation:** A homeopathic formulation used for relief from symptoms of constipation.

☐ **Nature's Way Primadophilus:** A supplement that helps restore a healthy bacterial population to the colon.

☐ **Yerba Prima Fiberdophilus:** A supplement that helps restore a healthy bacterial population to the colon.

☐ **Nature's Way Fiber Cleanse:** An herbal combination that is used to help relieve diarrheal problems and cleanse the colon.

☐ **Energy Medicine Diarrhea:** A homeopathic formulation used for relief of the symptoms of diarrhea.

☐ **Yerba Prima Echinace:** Research shows that the Echinacea herb helps to combat infection.

- ☐ **Nature's Way Garlicin:** Research shows that garlic helps to combat infection.
- ☐ **Yerba Prima Chamomile:** An herb with properties that are calming and soothing to the digestive tract.
- ☐ **Energy Medicine Nausea (Vomiting):** A homeopathic formulation used for relief of the symptoms of nausea and vomiting.

Often, when constipation (difficult, infrequent defecation) occurs, our first impulse is to take a laxative. Forty million Americans currently use laxatives and eight million of these use them at least once a week![25] Unfortunately, once a laxative has passed through the colon, we usually find the bowels to be as sluggish as ever. With continued use, the bowel experiences poor muscle tone, faulty peristalsis (muscle movements of intestine wall that move fecal material along), and the result can be further dependence on laxatives. Even with all these negative affects, nothing has been done to remove the stagnant residue coating the intestine wall that contributes to the malfunctioning of the colon. Laxatives simply encourage the body to rely on laxatives and we find it becomes more and more difficult to have a normal bowel movement without the help of a purging agent.

There is a natural laxative herb called cascara sagrada that is reputed not only to have laxative action, but to tone and strengthen the bowels as well.[26] Because of this, some experts say you have a less likely chance of becoming dependent on cascara. This herb is said to possess many digestive benefits, some of which include the ability to increase secretions of the liver, stomach, pancreas, and the lower bowels.[27] The fresh bark should be avoided as it may produce nausea. As the herb ages from 1 to 6 years, however, oxidation takes place, and this preparation becomes milder and more effective as both a tonic and a laxative. This wonderful herb, which we inherited from the American Indians, produces large painless stools without cramping, and after extended usage, the bowels will be strengthened by its tonic effects.[28]

Both Nature's Way Cascara Sagrada and Nature's Herbs Cascara Sagrada are quality products. In some cases it may be advantageous to use this herb, but in general it is better to prevent the problem by maintaining a high-fiber diet and healthy intestinal flora. Psyllium husks, a high-fiber supplement mentioned earlier that's made from the dried seed coat of the *Plantago ovata* plant, will usually help in mild cases of constipation without your having to resort to a laxative. If you have developed a dependency on laxatives or just find irregularity to be a recurrent problem, what you probably need is a good cleansing regime to remove encrusted waste and improve the elimination system.

A homeopathic preparation for constipation is also available. Energy Medicine Constipation is produced by Dolisos America Inc. and is composed of five separate remedies that deal with the symptoms of constipation. This preparation has helped many who suffer from sluggish bowels and may be of benefit to you as well.

Diarrhea (frequent passage of watery bowel movements) can also be caused by this same problem of fecal deposits. Chronic diarrhea is often due to the presence of infection or irritation in the colon; in fact, this is how many laxatives function. The laxative creates an irritation that stimulates the bowel to empty itself. The unhealthy conditions that accompany old fecal deposits can lead to irritation and, in extreme conditions, diseases such as diverticulitis (small herniations through the muscular wall of the colon), colon cancer, and other serious conditions. A frightening fact to note: colon cancer is second only to lung cancer as the leading cause of cancer death.[29]

Short-lived diarrhea can also be induced by food poisoning, which some authorities state is much more common than most of us imagine.[30] Anxiety has also been recognized as another potential cause of diarrhea. The tendency of antibiotics to destroy and cause imbalance to the intestinal flora can also lead to diarrhea. Many medical authorities suggest supplementing antibiotic treatment with an acidophilus or bifidus product. An acidophilus supplement such as Nature's Way Primadophilus or Yerba Prima Fiberdophilus can help to restore the healthy bacterial population and may rectify this condition.

Many anti-diarrheal drugs have possible dangerous side effects such as numbness of extremities, depression, headaches, vomiting, and increased heart rate.[31] Some natural items that sometimes help reduce the number of bowel movements in the case of diarrhea include bananas, carob powder, and cinnamon. Black tea may offer some help if nothing else is available.

Remember to use caution in stopping the body processes from trying to rid itself of some kind of toxic substance. If we take too much of an anti-diarrheal agent we may stop our bowel movements prematurely and uncomfortable cramping may result. As long as diarrhea is not due to some more serious medical problem, it is best to let the condition run its course. Be sure to replace lost fluids and electrolytes by drinking plenty of warm water and honey. Dehydration can be a serious problem accompanying severe cases of diarrhea, especially in children.

Psyllium husks, the cleaned, dried seed coat gathered by winnowing and thrashing the seeds of the botanical, *Plantago ovata*, are rich in mucilage (a type of fiber source known as hemicellulose). Mucilage increases bulk in the intestines by retaining water. In the case of diarrhea, the absorption of excess water can help relieve this condition. Psyllium husks are the active ingredients of Nature's Way Fiber Cleanse, a product often used to cleanse the colon, but also helpful when dealing with diarrheal problems. Because it also contains fennel seed, which helps prevent cramping, it serves two functions when used for this condition.[32]

Energy Medicine Diarrhea formula from Dolisos offers relief to many for the discomfort of some simple diarrheal conditions. This homeopathic preparation is a combination of nine individual remedies. Energy Medicine Diarrhea is a formulation that may help relieve the discomfort of loose stools, but again, be cautious about halting such a condition too quickly, as your body may need to rid itself of toxic substances.

Echinacea or garlic (see Yerba Prima Echinace and Nature's Way Garlicin discussed in Chapter 5) will help combat any infection that may be present, and chamomile (see Yerba Prima Chamomile discussed earlier in this chapter) can help settle feelings of nausea. Speaking of nausea, there is a homeopathic preparation available for this uncomfortable problem, which I have already mentioned. Energy Medicine Nausea (Vomiting) is a combination of five homeopathics to aid the body's efforts to alleviate this unsettling condition.

Though these products may help bring needed relief for specific conditions, we need to look deeper and treat the factors causing these symptoms. Instead of only concentrating on what to take for constipation, diarrhea, or other problems associated with the large intestine, I feel that overall colon health needs our primary attention. When the colon is free of accumulations of old feces, irritation is less likely to occur, parasites cannot maintain a strong foothold in the body, and, because the colon can function properly, a normal transit time of fecal material should be a common occurrence.

Colon Cleansing Program

From my experience and research, the best way to bring an unhealthy colon to a state of health is with a good, fiber-based cleansing system. I already covered some of the basics on cleansing in Chapter 3. At this time I want to give you an example of a good cleansing program you can use without having to change your eating habits too drastically.

Some Natural Products for a Colon Cleansing Program:

- [ ] **Yerba Prima Internal Cleansing Program:** Consists of two products, Kalenite and Colon Care Formula, which help cleanse the colon as well as other body systems. **Yerba Prima Kalenite** is a blend of cleansing and purifying herbs for the entire digestive tract and for other organs and systems of the body. **Yerba Prima Colon Care Formula** offers a source of fiber, calcium, and beneficial intestinal bacteria.
- [ ] **Yerba Prima Vivalo Creme:** A moisturizing agent applied to the abdominal region to encourage the release of encrusted fecal matter and often used in conjunction with the Internal Cleansing Program.
- [ ] **Yerba Prima Aloe Vera Juice with Herbs:** An herbal juice that promotes a healthy bacterial population in the colon.

Just in case you think I am partial to the Yerba Prima Company, I am, at least as far as digestive products are concerned. For many years, this company has led the industry in this field and also was one of the first to bring some outstanding standardized herbal products to this country from Europe and other areas of the world. So why not give credit where credit is due?

I'm also not the only one who approves of the Yerba Prima Program. It is the chosen program in *Intestinal Toxicity and Inner Cleansing* by Dr. Jeffery Bland, and *Internal Cleansing: A Practical Guide to Colon Health* by Linda Berry, D.C., as well as a subject of a clinical study by the Linus Pauling Institute of Science and Medicine. Subjects in this study reported an improved feeling of well being, less frequency of headaches, and higher energy levels. In addition, it was found that individuals who participated in the program showed a reduction in harmful bacteria, an increase in vitamin absorption, and better protein absorption.[33] My own experience has shown this program is very gentle, very easy, and very effective.

Before describing the program, let me mention an important factor dealing with cleansing. This is the issue of cleansing reactions. If a cleansing regime is not begun gradually, the rapid release of stored toxins into the bloodstream faster than they can be eliminated can cause what is known as a cleansing reaction. These can occur as headaches, dizziness, disturbed sleep, emotional unrest, skin rashes, digestive upsets, gas, joint pains, and respiratory colds. Many people have shied away from natural cleansing programs because they feared these cleansing reactions. These reactions can be avoided or kept to a minimum if the cleansing formula is properly balanced, and the individual is careful to begin the program slowly. My experience with the Yerba Prima Program has proven it to be a very gentle approach to cleansing. Except for an occasional dip in energy level and/or a bloated feeling in the first few days, I have not seen any other negative effects in myself or other friends participating in the program.

The Yerba Prima Program is a complete cleansing system to be used as a preventative means to assist in keeping the entire body's elimination functions open and cleansed so they are able to accomplish their important functions. Proper elimination requires not only a clean colon, but also proper functioning of the kidneys, urinary tract, liver, gall bladder, lymphatic system, and the skin. So it is important for a cleansing system to assist all of these eliminative processes.

The Yerba Prima Program consists of two primary products. The first is Kalenite, an herbal tablet made up of a blend of cleansing and purifying herbs. This formula is designed to work with the body to naturally cleanse the liver, blood, lymphatic system, kidneys, colon, and entire gastrointestinal tract. Colon Care Formula, the second important constituent of the program, is a high-fiber formula capable of several functions. This formula includes a balance of soluble and insoluble fibers (psyllium husks, barley fiber, guar gum, oat bran, and fruit pectin), which contains all five fiber types (hemicellulose, gums or mucilages, pectin, cellulose, and lignin). For the most part, insoluble fibers like cellulose and lignin are considered to pass through the digestive system without being broken down. On the other hand, soluble fibers like pectin and gums are broken down. Hemicellulose tends to contain both insoluble and soluble qualities. The functions performed by these fiber types include absorbing and quickly removing toxins released into the colon, producing softer stools that are easy to eliminate from the body, helping to build a healthy bacterial population, and reducing pressure in the colon.

In addition to fiber, Colon Care Formula contains a high potency of the four most important beneficial bacteria contributing to colon health, all in a hypoallergenic, non-dairy culture, free of soy, yeast, wheat, milk, and eggs. This product contains no sugar, preservatives, colors, or artificial flavors. Colon Care Formula also includes two types of calcium: calcium carbonate and calcium citrate. Calcium helps the friendly bacteria pass through the stomach and provides nutritional support to the mucosal lining of the colon. Dr. Martin Lipkin, a researcher studying the effects of calcium on colon health, reports that evidence has shown calcium helps protect the colon in several ways. Increased calcium content of the epithelial cells reduces overly rapid cell growth, and unabsorbed calcium neutralizes irritating fatty acids and bile acids in the colon. In addition, free calcium in the colon buffers and protects the mucosa.[34] As research continues, more evidence supports the benefits of this element on colon health including a recent study concluding that people who consumed more calcium had less risk of developing colon cancer.[35]

Vivalo Creme, an olive oil moisturizer, which is applied topically to the abdominal region, is another product that can be used with this cleansing duet. Its primary function is to penetrate the walls of the colon in order to soften and release old, encrusted fecal matter.

This program is as simple as taking one to three tablets with a teaspoon of fiber in water a few times per day. After two weeks, if you wish, you can put the cream on your abdomen twice a day. No diet restraints are necessary, though it stands to reason that cleansing will be faster and more effective if you improve your diet while on the program. The program can be used daily, for up to five months, but from six to twelve weeks is considered optimum. Many repeat this regime once or twice a year to assure a long-term healthy elimination system.

There are a few other items to add to your cleansing program to assure even more benefits. The first is skin brushing, discussed at length in the section on cleaning procedures. Skin brushing can really aid in the elimination of excess toxins released during the cleansing process. The second item that can be added to your cleansing program is aloe vera juice. In addition to having a soothing and healing effect on the entire digestive tract, it promotes a healthy bacterial population. Two to four ounces of aloe juice per day for several weeks, at the beginning and after ending this cleansing regime, is especially beneficial. Yerba Prima puts out an excellent product under the name Aloe Vera plus Herbs.

Everyone suffers from time to time from some type of intestinal problem whether it be intestinal pain, flatulence, constipation, diarrhea, or bloating. Recurrence of these problems can lead to more serious conditions and should be a signal to participate in a cleansing program such as the one I have just described. I feel there is little reason to doubt that maintaining a clean and healthy colon will contribute significantly to a person's total health.

Liver Problems

Our largest organ, the liver, located in the upper right portion of the abdominal cavity, is reddish-brown in color, and weighs about three pounds. The importance of this organ cannot be stressed enough as it performs over 500 different functions. With only one-sixth of your liver intact, you could still function fairly normally, and if 80 percent of your liver was cut out, it could grow back to its original size in just three months! Because of its hardy design, it is difficult to determine whether a liver is damaged until the damage has become quite advanced.[36]

Some of the major functions of the liver include synthesizing blood proteins, Vitamin A, cholesterol, and glucose. Bile salts are also produced in the liver and secreted into the small intestine. These salts help to emulsify fat particles, neutralize intestinal acid, and remove toxins from the liver. Another function of the liver is the conversion of ammonia from the breakdown of proteins into urea for excretion by the kidneys. Filtering bacteria from the intestines so they will not enter the general bloodstream is still another chore the liver performs. A well-functioning liver will tone down blood sugar swings by up to 65 percent and can convert dietary fatty acids into circulating phospholipids for easier utilization by the cells.

Perhaps one of the most important functions of this organ is detoxification. The liver detoxifies incompletely digested proteins, excess hormones, drugs, food additives, poisons, and other substances that may cause a threat to the well-being of the body. It is capable of converting up to one-half ounce of alcohol into carbon dioxide and water in just one hour. I'm sure some "party animals" out there owe the lives of many a brain cell to our friend the liver.

The list of items that cause a threat to the health of the liver are the very things that this organ works so hard to protect us from. The elements threatening to the liver are really too numerous to list, but I will mention a few of the most obvious factors that have a detrimental effect on this organ. The most common cause of toxic liver damage is the excessive consumption of alcohol.[37] Fried foods, animal fats, hydrogenated fat, too much vegetable oil, and roasted nuts can congest the liver as well. Polluted air and water, strong cleaning solutions, strong medications, pesticides, herbicides, food additives, preservatives, drugs, birth control pills, nicotine, caffeine, too much protein, corticosteroids, refined sugar, and ferrous sulfate as an iron supplement can all overtax and cause damage to this vital organ. Nerve pressure in the mid-thoracic vertebrae of the back can also interfere with proper functioning of the liver. Another cause of liver dysfunction is a toxic colon, which has already been discussed in detail. So as you see, living a normal life in our modern society can inflict quite a beating on one of our most important organs.

As stated before, we may not realize we have an unhealthy liver until we are stricken with a serious illness. If we have gotten to the point of suffering from a serious liver ailment, we should definitely be in the hands of a qualified physician because such a condition is nothing to fool around with. Some of the more grave conditions include: cirrhosis (a degenerative disease), hepatitis (an inflammation of the liver), and jaundice (a yellow discoloration of the skin due to excess bile in the body fluids).

How do we prevent ending up with one of these less than desirable conditions? It is not always easy to change our habits. Our way of life has become so incorporated with technology and a fast pace of living, it is often difficult to focus on balancing it with a natural way of living. We have to take small steps at first, creating new beneficial habits, one at a time. First we can cut down our intake of alcohol and some of the other unhealthy foods listed above. We can also try to avoid frequent contact with strong cleaning solutions and other toxic chemicals we might encounter. We can increase the number of live foods (fresh fruits and vegetables) in our diet and add supplemental enzymes. And finally, a periodic cleansing of the liver can be of great benefit in maintaining the health of this important organ.

Some Natural Products Used for Improving Liver Function:

☐ **Yerba Prima LivCleanse:** Tablets containing milk thistle herb, which can improve the condition of the liver.

☐ **Nature's Way Thisilyn:** Capsules containing milk thistle herb, which can improve the condition of the liver.

☐ **Kyolic Aged Garlic Extract:** Research shows that aged garlic extract can aid the liver by removing toxic substances from the body.

☐ **Rainbow Light All-Zyme:** An herbal supplement that contains all four food enzyme groups and acts as an enzyme replacement and digestive aid.

☐ **Floradix Herbal Bitters:** An herbal formula that promotes liver function and increases bile secretion.

There are several regimes that one can follow to cleanse the liver. One, known as the liver flush, combines cold-pressed olive oil (2 tablespoons), the juice of fresh-squeezed citrus fruit (1 lemon and 1–2 oranges), and crushed garlic (1–4 cloves). This concoction is mixed in a blender and then drunk, followed by two cups of hot tea, each morning for ten to twelve days. Afterwards, no other food except citrus fruit should be eaten for two hours. If a healthy diet accompanies your liver flush regime, your liver and gall bladder can be cleansed significantly.

Fortunately, today there are excellent herbal products available that can make this complicated process quite a bit more simple. Yerba Prima has still another product known as Yerba Prima LivCleanse. This product contains only one herbal ingredient, the milk thistle seed (*Silybum marianum*), which has been consumed since the time of ancient Greece and is still used by millions of people the world over for its health and nutritional benefits. Over forty years of scientific research has been done in Europe on the milk thistle seed. The nutritive ingredient in milk thistle is silymarin and together with its essential components, are standardized in LivCleanse tablets in quantities to assure optimal benefits (70 milligrams per tablet/1–2 tablets, three times per day).

In Germany, scientific studies show that the action of silymarin consists of the protection of intact liver cells and the stimulation of protein synthesis, which accounts for an increase of new cells. Studies also show that silymarin benefits the kidneys.[38] Further proof of the effectiveness of silymarin is found in a study involving 97 patients in Helsinki, Finland, all of which exhibited elevated serum transaminase levels. High levels of the liver enzyme transaminase are indicative of liver damage.[39] Blood and histological tests were performed before and at the completion of the study. After four weeks with one group on 420 milligrams per day of silymarin and the other on a placebo, the researchers stated: "Improvement of morphological alterations occurred significantly more often in the silymarin-treated group. Because these determinants of liver disease are methodologically unrelated and represent substantially different aspects of the state of the liver, it is probable that their improvement can be ascribed to real improvement in the state of the liver."[40] In other words, many of the subjects who took the silymarin daily showed signs that the health of their livers had improved.

Another study by a European phytochemist named Dr. Vogel showed amazing effects from silymarin when used to treat poisoning from the death cup mushroom (*Amanita phalloides*), which has the capacity to destroy liver tissue. Dr. Vogel found silymarin could regenerate liver cells already compromised, as well as prevent the toxin from reaching healthy cell membranes. In addition, studies have determined no toxic effects from milk thistle, except for occasional loose stools when excessive amounts are taken.[41]

Another high quality milk thistle extract is available from Nature's Way. Each Nature's Way Thisilyn capsule contains 140 milligrams of silymarin. The European company that produces Thisilyn for Nature's Way breeds their plants for the highest concentration of silymarin, and then carefully monitors the extraction process. In addition, they analyze the extract to ensure that it retains all the desired natural benefits of the milk thistle plant.

The LivCleanse tablets and Thisilyn capsules are simple to use and many people feel results in a very short time. It is ideal to be able to withdraw the liver-damaging agents from our diet and environment, but it is not always possible. In these cases, it is valuable to know that milk thistle seed will reliably reverse toxic hepatic dysfunctions of different origins.[42] If you have completed the internal cleansing program described previously, you might want to follow it with a couple of weeks of liver cleansing. Or if you just want to be kind to your liver, Liv-Cleanse and Thisilyn are both wonderful products.

One other supplement known for its remarkable detoxifying properties is Kyolic Aged Garlic Extract. Kyolic has been the subject of numerous clinical and laboratory research projects and has been shown to remove toxic chemicals from the body. Back in 1975, the *Journal of Food Science* reported that aged garlic extract added to the diet was able to counteract the toxic effects of the artificial food coloring agents FD and C Red No. 2 (amaranth), FD and C Blue No. 1 (brilliant blue), and FD and C Violet. A 5 percent addition of these coloring agents to the diets of animals resulted in diarrhea, low body weight, and a lack of normal grooming patterns. These adverse effects completely disappeared when the animals were also given aged garlic extract.[43] Kyolic Aged Garlic Extract has been shown to remove organic chemicals from the body, as well as heavy metals.[44] Any agent that can help the liver in its overwhelming chore of cleansing the body of toxic substances deserves consideration when trying to improve the health of this valuable organ. This product will be discussed in more detail in Chapter 5.

The presence of enzymes in your food can have an effect on the health of the liver. In the upper portion of the stomach, known as the fundic region, no digestive enzymes are secreted. It is in this area where salivary enzymes and the enzymes found naturally in foods act to initially break down the food we have eaten.[45] In this way, some of the digestive process gets performed before the food is moved on to the enzyme-secreting area of the stomach and the intestines. Enzymes are completely destroyed by exposure to heat above 129°F.[46] This means that there are virtually no live enzymes available in cooked foods. When we eat a diet of predominantly cooked foods over a period of many years, it eliminates the usefulness of this predigestion process. This, in turn, allows for putrefaction of foodstuffs that add toxins to the blood stream. It also causes the digestive organs to work harder to provide enzymes for the digestive processes.

Amylase is an enzyme that breaks down starch and is found in many live foods that contain starch. In an experiment involving forty patients with liver diseases such as cirrhosis, hepatitis, and cholecystitis, all showed low levels of blood amylase. But when there was a rise in the blood amylase level, there was an improvement in the general condition of each patient, as well as an improvement in liver function.[47] Perhaps 80 percent of diseases are caused by improperly digested foods and their byproducts being absorbed into the body.[48] I'm not trying to suggest that you exist on raw foods, but if you eat a quantity of foods containing active enzymes, such as sprouts and fruit, or if you take supplemental enzymes, it can be beneficial and may even extend the health of your liver as well as some other important organs.

Rainbow Light All-Zyme is an enzyme supplement that was discussed earlier in this chapter. All-Zyme contains all four food enzyme groups, including amylase, and acts as an enzyme replacement and digestive aid. The use of this supplement could help reduce the quantity of digestive enzymes the liver normally must produce, and therefore, aid in maintaining a healthier liver.

Another supplement that promotes liver function is Floradix Herbal Bitters, already mentioned in detail when I talked about digestive aids earlier in this chapter. This product, when taken at meal time, especially when indulging in rich foods, will encourage the necessary bile secretion needed to digest the additional fats.

5

The Respiratory System

Every cell in our bodies needs a continuous supply of oxygen for metabolic activities, as well as the constant removal of the carbon dioxide waste product of this metabolism. The tissues depend on the respiratory system for maintaining our lives by carrying out these essential functions. The transportation of these gases between the cells and the respiratory system is accomplished by the circulatory system. The respiratory system helps in the exchange of these important gases between the external environment and the blood circulating through the lungs. Here, excess carbon dioxide is released and needed oxygen is drawn in.

A secondary function related to the respiratory system is the regulation of acid-base (pH) balance in the blood. Because carbon dioxide is acidic, the blood becomes overly acidic when there is excess carbon dioxide present. Conversely, if too little carbon dioxide is present in the blood, it can become overly alkaline. The rate and depth of our breaths serve to regulate the amount of carbon dioxide in our blood within a very narrow range of concentrations.[1]

Since the specific purpose of the respiratory tract is to bring air close enough to the blood to allow the exchange of oxygen and carbon dioxide, a passage to the exterior is necessary. The upper respiratory tract, consisting of the nose, pharynx, larynx, trachea, and the bronchi, forms an open passageway between the lungs and the exterior. The lungs are the main organs of respiration. The right lung consists of three lobes, the left lung two. Their extensive network of capillaries provides adequate surface area for a high rate of exchange of these gases.

The intercostal muscles of the chest and the muscular diaphragm provide the mechanical force to fill and empty the lungs in the process we know as breathing. During inspiration, the diaphragm moves downward and the lungs expand, filling with air. During expiration, the diaphragm moves upward again, forcing the air out. We normally have a respiratory rate of about sixteen breaths per minute. The amount of oxygen we need during heavy exercise can be as much as twenty times more than the need when we are resting. When we're healthy, our respiratory rate adapts accordingly.

As breathing occurs, air enters through the nose and mouth and travels down the trachea towards the lungs. At the point where the trachea enters the lungs, it branches out into bronchi and then into smaller bronchioles and eventually into 250 million air sacs called alveoli. It is here in the alveoli, rich in capillaries, that the exchange of oxygen and carbon dioxide takes place. The interior surface of the lung is by far the most extensive body surface in contact with the environment, its area being many times greater than that of the skin.[2]

When our body gets overloaded and needs to release unwanted waste products, our respiratory system can act as an organ of elimination. Uncomfortable respiratory ailments such as the common cold, flu, allergies, and bronchial problems may be symptoms of problems in this elimination function. We will now look at some products that have provided relief for many sufferers of these ailments.

Colds and Flu

The immune system consists of several different elements of the body. When strong and functioning properly, it protects our body from many common ailments. The standard American diet has left most of our immune systems in sad shape indeed. Attention to nutrition can help to reverse this trend and allow our body defenses to work at their optimum.

I have included the discussion of the immune system with the discussion of the respiratory system because the latter is so often affected by symptoms such as colds and flu during times of lowered resistance. Please be aware, however, that the respiratory system is not the only system in the body that offers immune mechanisms. Many other systems and organs of the body contribute to and are affected by the strength of our immune functions.

The spleen, a major organ of the immune system, assists in the production of white blood cells that attack viral and bacterial intruders. In Chinese medicine, the function of the stomach and pancreas in digestion are considered to be related directly to the spleen; these two are the first organs to be treated in order to bolster immune function.[3] Proper digestion enhanced by proper diet is considered the first step in assuring a strong immune response.

Because the immune system is a primary player in the network of body defenses, when it is functioning optimally, often the common ailments of colds and flu do not infect us. Doesn't it seem strange that when a "bug" is going around, some people are affected and others seem to be able to ward it off? Perhaps the defenses of these so-called "immune" individuals are just stronger. When our resistance is down due to stress, lack of sleep, or improper diet, we are usually more prone to contracting an illness.

Indications of the effects of stress on resistance to disease were studied in-depth by researchers of Mount Sinai School of Medicine in New York City. They found that two months after the death of spouses, widowers suffered a depressed immune function. It seems that during stressful times, the body releases large quantities of a steroid known as *cortisol*, which limits the ability of macrophages (white blood cells that engulf foreign particles in the blood stream) to respond normally to infection.[4] Other researchers, medical students at Ohio State University College of Medicine, found that subjects increased production of T-cells (cells that alert the body to impending invaders) after taking relaxation training.[5] So if stress is a factor in your life, you should take some measures to reduce the cause or learn techniques to cope with this stress, as well as take supplements to help strengthen your body's resistance to illness and disease.

There are some common vitamins and minerals that are known to be involved with immune functions. Vitamin A is especially important in helping to keep parts of the body that first come in contact with invading organisms strong, namely the skin and linings of the respiratory, digestive, and urogenital tracts, and the eyes. Vitamin A also enhances the B-cells, producers of plasma cells, which, in turn, manufacture antibodies.[6] Some research suggests that beta carotene is the preferred supplement for getting your required Vitamin A, because the body can better utilize and assimilate it in this form.

Some of the B-complex vitamins are also involved in immune responses. Vitamins B-1, B-2, B-6, B-12, and folic acid are all important to immune function. Vitamin C is a well-known immune enhancer, made famous by Linus Pauling, Ph.D. in his book *Vitamin C, the Common Cold, and the Flu*. Vitamins D and E are also very important to the immune system, but some research has shown that too much of either of these can actually suppress immune-system effectiveness.[7]

Two minerals that are necessary for proper immune function are zinc and selenium. Zinc is a co-factor in more than 100 enzymes and its deficiency can lead to a reduction in the number of T-cells.[8] Selenium is an antioxidant, protecting cell walls from oxidation. In addition, selenium works with Vitamin E, enhancing the power of this important vitamin.

Some Natural Products Used for Flu and Cold Symptoms:

☐ **Boiron Borneman Oscillococcinum**: A homeopathic formulation used for the treatment of cold and flu symptoms (best used at the first signs of cold or flu).

☐ **Energy Medicine Flu Solution:** A homeopathic formulation used for the treatment of cold and flu symptoms (best used at the first signs of cold or flu).

☐ **Energy Medicine Influenza/Cold:** A homeopathic formulation used for the treatment of cold and flu symptoms (best used after cold or flu has set in).

☐ **Boericke & Tafel Alpha CF:** A homeopathic formulation containing no animal products and used for the treatment of cold and flu symptoms (used both at first signs and after cold or flu symptoms appear).

☐ **Zand Insure Herbal:** An herbal formula containing echinacea and goldenseal and used as a nutritional supplement for the immune system.

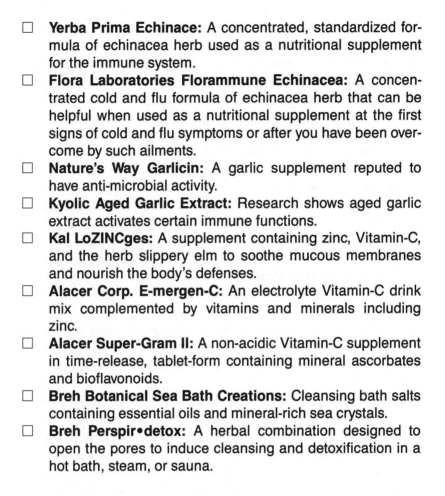

- ☐ **Yerba Prima Echinace:** A concentrated, standardized formula of echinacea herb used as a nutritional supplement for the immune system.
- ☐ **Flora Laboratories Florammune Echinacea:** A concentrated cold and flu formula of echinacea herb that can be helpful when used as a nutritional supplement at the first signs of cold and flu symptoms or after you have been overcome by such ailments.
- ☐ **Nature's Way Garlicin:** A garlic supplement reputed to have anti-microbial activity.
- ☐ **Kyolic Aged Garlic Extract:** Research shows aged garlic extract activates certain immune functions.
- ☐ **Kal LoZINCges:** A supplement containing zinc, Vitamin-C, and the herb slippery elm to soothe mucous membranes and nourish the body's defenses.
- ☐ **Alacer Corp. E-mergen-C:** An electrolyte Vitamin-C drink mix complemented by vitamins and minerals including zinc.
- ☐ **Alacer Super-Gram II:** A non-acidic Vitamin-C supplement in time-release, tablet-form containing mineral ascorbates and bioflavonoids.
- ☐ **Breh Botanical Sea Bath Creations:** Cleansing bath salts containing essential oils and mineral-rich sea crystals.
- ☐ **Breh Perspir•detox:** A herbal combination designed to open the pores to induce cleansing and detoxification in a hot bath, steam, or sauna.

There are some products that I have found to be quite effective in providing the nutrition needed to strengthen our system of body defenses. When those first symptoms of cold, flu, or lowered resistance start to appear, I reach for the herbal or homeopathic preparations that I have seen reverse the course towards ill health. More times than not, early dosages of specific products seemed to protect me while others were falling prey to the "bug" that was going around.

There are several products that I feel are especially impressive in their abilities to strengthen the body and therefore promote resistance to colds and flu. The first is Oscillococcinum, a homeopathic preparation derived from the heart and liver of

the *Anas Barbariae* duck, and manufactured by Boiron Borneman, Inc., a world leader in homeopathy. This product, with
thirty years of clinical research behind it, is the best-selling
product for flu-like symptoms in France, claiming almost half of
the market. It is also known to achieve more than a 90 percent
satisfaction factor from its consumers, an impressive figure
indeed![9]

In one recent study written up in the *British Journal of Clinical
Pharmacology*, researchers found that patients receiving Oscillococcinum for the treatment of influenza-like symptoms recovered within 48 hours, almost twice as fast as the group given a
placebo. The study is considered significant because of the
large sampling involved: 478 patients and 149 physicians participated. Most of the doctors were not homeopathic physicians
and neither doctor nor patient knew who received placebos and
who received the test medicine. Also, neither group knew it
was a homeopathic that was being tested.[10]

The makers of Oscillococcinum suggest it works best when
taken very soon after flu-like symptoms appear. Therefore, it is
a good idea to keep some around the house for the next time
you start coming down with the flu. As with other homeopathic remedies, doses should be taken at least fifteen minutes
before or one hour after eating. As soon as symptoms of fevers,
chills, body aches, and pains appear, dissolve the contents of a
tube under the tongue. Repeat this dose three times at six-hour
intervals.[11] As with other homeopathics, it acts gently to stimulate your natural defense mechanisms. I have seen some amazing results with this product.

Another, more economically-priced homeopathic product,
Energy Medicine Flu Solution by Dolisos America, is also available. Dolisos is the second largest company in France, second
only to Boiron. Perhaps my only problem with Oscillococcinum
is that it seems a bit overpriced. Also made from *Anas Barbariae*
duck liver and heart in a similar potency, Energy Medicine Flu
Solution seems to be identical to Oscillococcinum. Even though
the Flu Solution does not have the research record of the Oscillococcinum, from all indications and my personal experience,
the Dolisos product seems to work as well as the Boiron product. Priced at a considerable amount less than that of Oscillo-

coccinum, Energy Medicine Flu Solution seems to be a better value.

Both of these products are for use at the very first signs of lowered resistance and body aches and pains. There is also a homeopathic formula many use *after* a cold or flu-type illness has set in. Energy Medicine Influenza/Cold is a combination of eight remedies that often help the body combat some of the uncomfortable symptoms of unwelcome invaders that cause colds and flu.

One other homeopathic preparation to combat cold and flu symptoms is Boericke & Tafel Alpha CF tablets. First introduced in Holland, this remedy presently outsells any other cold and flu remedies in that country.[12] This product differs from other brands mentioned above in that it does not contain any animal by-products. For those who consider this an important factor, I have included it. Alpha CF can be used at the first signs of cold or flu or after these conditions have set in. Because it is a homeopathic, it contains no synthetic drugs, antihistamines, or vasoconstrictors. This medicinal preparation offers relief for sneezing, stuffy nose, coughing, chills, headache, fever, and the overall minor aches and pains that accompany those unwelcome "bugs."[13]

Three other products that I have found quite reliable for strengthening the system, especially when those first signs of lowered resistance start to become apparent, are each preparations using the herb echinacea. Echinacea, dating back to its use by the American Indians, was one of the primary medical agents of the past century. The herb was used to treat common fevers and minor infections, as well as other ailments like typhoid, meningitis, malaria, and diptheria. In the early 1930s, a German doctor named Dr. Madaus returned to Germany from North America with samples of the plant. For sixty years the Madaus Company has been doing extensive research and testing, and has continued developing methods for growing, harvesting, and processing echinacea.

Laboratory studies have shown that echinacea increases the ability of white blood cells to surround and destroy bacterial and viral invaders in the blood.[14] It also stimulates the lymphatic system to remove toxins and waste materials.[15] Echinacea destroys the germs of infection directly, bolsters the body's defenses by increasing the white blood cell count, and tends to normalize the temperature of the body.[16]

Recent research has discovered one of echinacea's mechanisms used to prevent infection. A substance known as hyaluronic acid (HA) is found in the tissues between the cells and acts as an effective barrier against infection. Hyaluronidase, an enzyme contained in certain bacteria, weakens HA and allows pathogenic bacteria, such as staph and strep, to penetrate the tissues and make you ill.[17] Echinacea has been shown to inhibit this enzyme activity, preventing the loss of HA and, therefore, raising cellular resistance.[18]

Because of its properties, echinacea extracts have been used extensively in hospitals and general practice in Europe. It is most widely used as a preventive measure for colds, flu, and upper respiratory conditions. It also maintains a place in the treatment of chronic health problems where the immune system needs strengthening.[19]

The three echinacea products I have had excellent success with are Zand Insure Herbal by Zand Herbal Formulas, Echinace by Yerba Prima, and Florammune Echinacea by Flora Laboratories. The Zand product contains both the roots of echinacea and goldenseal. Zand Herbal Formulas use a method known as the Dual Extraction Process to insure that both the alcohol and water-soluble substances are maximized. This allows for a wide range of active and bioavailable compounds to be extracted from the roots. Goldenseal has long been reported in botanical texts for its antibiotic action. The alkaloids of goldenseal, especially berberine and hydrastine, have been used to fight a wide variety of infectious agents.[20] The extracts of echinacea and goldenseal are combined in an herbal base of red clover, sage, burdock root, ginger, peppermint, parsley, fennel, chamomile, skullcap, bayberry, cayenne, valerian, and barberry. This formulation was created by Dr. Janet Zand, a well-known naturopath, who uses herbal medicine, homeopathy, nutrition, and acupuncture in her practice. She has treated thousands of patients with an impressive improvement success rate of over 90 percent.[21] The recommended dosage is 15–20 drops every two hours. Several people have reported to me that they have often found positive results after taking 15 drops every hour (for 3–4 hours) when those first symptoms of lowered resistance appear. I have experienced the same impressive results.

Zand Insure Herbal was previously called Zand Immune Herbal. Recently, the FDA asked many herbal and nutritional companies to remove the word "immune" from their labels. Because there have been no immune-related guidelines for the use of prescription or over-the-counter (OTC) products, and because the FDA considers the use of the word "immune" a drug claim, they consider such claims illegal. Despite extensive foreign research on herbs such as echinacea and goldenseal, the FDA does not consider studies outside the United States as valid in determining new OTC guidelines. Consequently, many herbal formulas are sold as "food supplements," restricted by the FDA from mentioning benefits and conditions for use. In addition, the FDA is requesting that companies refrain from citing medical research and literature referring to the influence of these herbs on the immune system.[22] I understand that this paranoia with the term "immune" has to do with recent pressure groups wanting the FDA to work more quickly at legalizing potential AIDS medicines. It is truly a shame that the citizens of this country are being denied legitimate information with which to make their own educated decisions on the value and safety of their medicinals!

Echinace, an excellent product by Yerba Prima, has been grown and produced using highly refined methods. It is a potentized herbal extract made from 100 percent pure cold-pressed juice of freshly harvested, organically grown echinacea purpurea herbs. In this instance, "potentized" means that besides containing the entire echinacea herb, some of the isolated, active ingredients have also been added to assure that optimum levels of these substances exist in the finished product. Yerba's recommended dosage for Echinace is 20–40 drops, three times a day. I have found that, as with the Zand product, when one starts to feel lowered resistance, taking repeated doses every hour will often strengthen one's resistance to upper respiratory ailments.

Still another excellent echinacea product is Florammune Echinacea produced by Flora Laboratories. This product contains a blend of the two most effective echinacea species, *E. angustifolia* and *E. purpurea*. Both are organically grown in their natural habitat, North America, by Trout Lake Farms, one of the largest suppliers of certified organic herbs in the United States. The flowers, seeds, and roots are harvested separately, when each is at its optimum potential. Within minutes of harvest, with the use of a mobile laboratory that can be taken right into the field, the live echinacea plant is placed in natural pure grain alcohol for extraction, assuring its freshness.

Flora Laboratories has taken great care about doing the appropriate research and having the proper combination of herbs to achieve this potent formula. They went to the trouble to make the product and their facilities compliant with FDA regulations and are able to advertise Florammune Echinacea as a cold and flu formula directly on their label. My experience has shown that this product can be helpful when used either at the first signs of cold and flu symptoms or after you have been overcome by such ailments.

All these products may help your body fight off a "bug" or possibly reduce the period you suffer with cold or flu-like symptoms if taken after the symptoms occur. They may also help strengthen your defenses when taken in a preventative manner. Many people take one of these products when cold and flu season starts just to increase their chances of avoiding these undesirable influences. All are available in both tablet and liquid form, but the liquid is generally considered quite a bit more potent.

Another herb that should be mentioned in regard to strengthening the system is garlic. Garlic was a treasured medicine of the ancient Egyptians, East Indians, Chinese, Hebrews, Babylonians, Vikings, Phoenicians, Greeks, and Romans. Hippocrates used this herb to treat pneumonia and pus-forming wounds. When Columbus arrived in the "New World," he discovered the American Indians harvesting garlic. It was also utilized in World War I to prevent gangrene and was known in World War II as "Russian Penicillin."

Today, we know that garlic prevents colds and fevers by increasing resistance to infection and stress; it's also extremely nutritious.[23] Garlic contains high levels of Vitamins A and C, thiamine, protein, and trace elements of aluminum, calcium, copper, germanium, iron, potassium, selenium, sulfur, tin, and zinc. Garlic works as an antibiotic against bacterial and fungal agents that cause a number of ailments.

Allicin, a compound acknowledged to provide much of garlic's antibacterial and antifungal activity, has been studied extensively.[24] One milligram of allicin is estimated to equal the strength of fifteen standard units of penicillin![25] Findings of two independent researchers in Japan and Romania determined that garlic is able to protect living organisms from the flu virus.[26] Even though allicin can be a helpful aid to the body defenses, there is also evidence that in large quantities it can have some detrimental influences. Thirty grams per day of raw garlic, lightly cooked garlic, or garlic juice can cause burns to the mouth, esophagus, and stomach as well as contribute to anemia and other conditions.[27] For this reason, it is inadvisable to supplement the diet with the large quantities of fresh garlic that are required to be effective against disease.

There are quite a few garlic products available on the supplement shelves of natural foods stores. Most are processed to eliminate the odor associated with garlic, much of which is caused by the allicin in the fresh product. Though many of these products seem to be good vehicles of some of the health-giving properties of fresh garlic, one product that I have confidence in is produced by Nature's Way. Nature's Way Garlicin seems to show a closer resemblance to fresh garlic than its competitors. Nature's Way first uses three technical processes to extract the important ingredients. Then, instead of using processes to remove the garlic odor (including much of the allicin, which is very unstable at room temperature,[28] the company coats the product so it can proceed to the intestines before being digested. This prevents the bounceback of flavor and odor from the stomach that non-coated products may induce.[29]

Though fresh garlic and Garlicin show superior antimicrobial properties in some research studies—that is, the ability to destroy detrimental microbes—another product exhibits its own beneficial properties. About thirty-five years ago, Wakunaga Pharmaceutical of Japan developed a natural cold-aging process that produces an odorless aged garlic called Kyolic. Kyolic Aged Garlic Extract, the subject of many research studies, provides not only many of the usual benefits of fresh garlic, but also many new benefits.[30] While protecting the body from certain infections, it does not exert its effects directly on the microbes as antibiotics or the allicin in fresh garlic do. Kyolic activates the immunoresponder cells (including macrophages), increases the natural killer cell activity (another of our immune system allies), and has been shown to protect mice from infection by the influenza virus.[31,32]

Besides allicin, garlic is rich in biological sulfhydryl compounds and polysulfides. Dr. Robert I-San Lin states in his book *Garlic in Nutrition and Medicine* that these compounds can stimulate immune function. There have even been tests on AIDS patients conducted by a Florida pathologist, Dr. Tariq Abdullah, that have shown the ability of Kyolic Aged Garlic Extract to improve immune functions. In these tests, natural killer cell activity was measured because AIDS patients commonly have drastically decreased natural killer cell activity. But after only six weeks on aged odorless garlic, about 90 percent of the patients had their natural killer cell activity returned to normal.[33] Symptoms of diarrhea, genital herpes, Candida albicans infections, and pansinusitis with fever also showed improvement.[34]

As we age our immune functions gradually lose their strength and their ability to defend us against disease. For this reason Kyolic Aged Garlic Extract can be an excellent supplement to consider adding to our diets. Four Kyolic capsules are equivalent to approximately two ounces of fresh garlic. To take this much fresh garlic could be toxic due to the high amounts of allicin present.[35] As mentioned before, however, research indicates that large amounts of raw garlic can cause anemia, as well as burning and irritation to the intestinal tract.[36] Also, the pungent odor that your body would emit from taking so much raw garlic would discourage most people from coming near you—hence, discouraging you from taking such large quantities! In tests conducted by Dr. Lin, dose levels of Kyolic given to animals equivalent to 100 times the recommended human dose level demonstrated no side effects.[37]

Kyolic Aged Garlic Extract is available in two standard forms. Don't be confused by all the different formulations of this product line. Some contain other nutrients, such as Vitamin B-1 and magnesium, to further enhance specific usages. Basically, you can purchase this product in dry tablets, dry capsules, or in liquid. In addition, the liquid can be obtained by itself or with empty capsules for enclosing the liquid. I strongly recommend the liquid form because it seems more potent and effective than the dry form of the herb. Some people like to squirt some of the liquid into the mouth and follow it with a glass of water. This practice usually leaves a bit of garlic odor in the mouth for about five minutes. Others who dislike the garlic taste, prefer to fill the capsules and ingest it this way. (When you purchase Kyolic with empty capsules, the handy container makes filling the capsules very easy without being messy.) Whatever your preference, Kyolic offers wonderful nutritional support to your body's defense network.

One supplement many find helpful during cold and flu season is Kal LoZINCges. These LoZINCges contain zinc aspartate (a palatable form of zinc), a pH-balanced form of Vitamin C for general health and healing, and Vitamin A, vital for the mucous membranes and respiratory system. This product also contains the herb slippery elm, originally used by the American Indians and known for its ability to soothe the mucous membranes.[38]

Many people like to load up on Vitamin C when threatened by colds or flu. Vitamin C is known to provide countless benefits to the human body because it is involved in so many bodily functions. Part of the list is: skin flexibility and health, adrenaline production, serotonin production (the chemical messenger of the brain), prevention of plaque formation in the arteries and veins, detoxification of the body, protection from pollution, wound healing, and the strengthening of immune functions.[39] If you are looking for a good Vitamin-C supplement, my recommendation would have to be Alacer Corp. E-mergen-C. This outstanding product combines a variety of mineral and vitamin supplements, including zinc, to complement the effects of Vitamin C. The powdered formula comes in a handy, pre-measured packet, which can be dissolved in cold water to provide a refreshing drink.

Vitamin C, being both an electron donor and an electron acceptor, has the ability to enter into countless chemical reactions in the body. It is a very unstable substance, especially as ascorbic acid, and therefore tends to link up with any other charged body it comes in contact with. The only form in which it is circulated or stored in the human body is as a mineral ascorbate.[40] (A mineral ascorbate is the form Vitamin C takes when combined with a mineral.) Some examples are calcium ascorbate, zinc ascorbate, and magnesium ascorbate. In this form, Vitamin C and the mineral with which it is combined can move to any part of the body where it is needed and can easily be transported into the cells. It is in this ascorbate form that E-mergen-C offers us our Vitamin C supplementation.

Many athletes also use E-mergen-C to restore electrolytes and other substances that can be depleted with heavy exercise. It is preferred by health-conscious individuals because it is free of additives and contains less salt and more potassium (eight times more than the sports drink called Gatorade) to keep the body's delicate sodium/potassium ratio in balance.

Still another Vitamin C supplement by Alacer Corp. is Alacer Super-Gram II. This product is similar to E-mergen-C, but it contains its nutrients, including 1,000 milligrams of Vitamin C, in time-release tablet form for those who prefer this method of supplementation. This non-acidic formula consists of five neutral, mineral ascorbates, which are readily assimilated sources of both Vitamin C and minerals, as well as eight bioflavonoids. Bioflavonoids are co-factors that are found with natural forms of Vitamin C and assist in its health-giving actions.

Super-Gram II is a large tablet, though not as large as some tablets I've seen. Just a little tip for those that have difficulty swallowing tablets or capsules, especially the larger ones. Hold the tablet against the roof of your mouth with your tongue and take two gulps of water. On the first gulp, only allow water to go down your throat, but release the tablet or capsule on the second gulp. How does this help? There is a shelf-like structure above the vocal cords known as the epiglottis, which must fold down to allow material to be swallowed. The first gulp of water stimulates it to fold down so that the pill can easily slide down on the second gulp.

Other techniques that may help relieve, shorten, or prevent cold- or flu-like conditions may be used with these products. One of the best methods I know to release toxins is to produce a sweat. The reason we get a fever is precisely for this purpose. The body defenses, attempting to eliminate toxic substances, heat up to push these unwanted invaders through the pores. A good hot bath with some quality bath salts to draw excess toxins through the skin not only helps the body in its cleansing, but also relieves the aches and pains often associated with these conditions. Breh Botanical Sea Bath Creations are my favorite bath salts. The Breh Company is devoted to making products with natural ingredients. They use only the purest essential oils and herbal extracts along with mineral-rich sea crystals and vegetable-based moisturizers. Sea water cleanses the skin of stale perspiration and impurities that block the pores, releases toxins and poisons from the skin, and has a rejuvenating and health-restoring effect.[41]

Breh's three original formulas, sandalwood, rose, and lavender, all contain the healing herbs comfrey and elder as well as the moisturizing properties of vegetable glycerin. The company also produces specialized bath formulas for specific health concerns, some of which I will be telling you about in upcoming chapters. I have tried many different bath salts over the years and have never found any to give the results I can obtain from these high-quality formulations. Usually about a half a cup of bath salts is enough for a single bath. It is advisable to drink a cup or two of hot tea before entering the bath. This will help to warm the body so perspiration will occur more easily, as well as add fluids to replace those expelled during the process.

I also use an herbal tincture of yarrow, elder flowers, and peppermint to add to my cup of tea to induce more sweat. At one time, I had marketed this combination as Sauna Tincture. Because of its concentration, Sauna Tincture was very easy to use. All you needed to do was add three drops to a cup of hot tea twenty minutes before getting into a sauna, hot tub, or bath. A tea made from these three dry herbs, if the herbs are of good quality, can also be effective in generating a good sweat. The first two herbs help to open the pores and the peppermint allows the other herbs to work a little more quickly.

One day I was talking to Charles Ames, the president of Breh Laboratories, about developing a product similar to Sauna Tincture to complement their line of bath salts. I offered him my formula just because I wanted the availability of such a product and was not interested in getting into the manufacturing business myself. After some research, Charles developed Breh Perspir•detox, designed to assist the detoxification process through perspiration. A few drops of this formula taken in hot tea just before stepping into a hot tub, bath, steam, or sauna can really enhance the cleansing process. The pore-opening properties of Perspir•detox, combined with the drawing effects of a quality bath salt, are capable of increasing the body's ability to rid itself of toxins through the skin.

People are always talking about finding the cure for the common cold. It we eat properly and use good sound herbal supplements to strengthen our natural systems of defense, we may suffer cold or flu-like symptoms less frequently. Or if we do fall prey to such nuisances, at least we might reduce the discomfort and the length of time we need to experience these circumstances. At any rate, I feel some of the products mentioned in this chapter should be available in the home and experimented with when we feel, due to lower resistance, "that cold coming on." I start taking one of the homeopathic preparations and one of the herbal formulas I have mentioned when those first signs of cold or flu show up. Of course, due to the delicate nature of the homeopathics, I take them at separate times. I've also been able to ward off many an illness with these products, even when too busy to slow down. If cold or flu symptoms have already taken hold, there are still other products that may be helpful in the reading that follows.

Remember that the change of the seasons in the fall and radical temperature changes at other times of the year can add stress to the system and may result in cold or flu-like symptoms. At these times, nutritional support can be especially important as a preventative measure.

Sinus Congestion

Maybe one of the most annoying problems associated with cold and flu-like symptoms is sinus congestion. Never being able to take a really full breath can be physically wearing. It's also no picnic having a tender nose as you go through your second box of tissues. Not to mention the painful experience of swollen sinuses. As I've mentioned before, I believe in treating uncomfortable symptoms, but in an intelligent way, with safe, effective agents. I also strongly recommend staying away from dairy products during these periods as they tend to be mucus-forming to many individuals and may cause increased congestion. Cigarette smoke and other irritating substances should also be avoided.

Some Natural Products Used for Sinus Congestion:

- ☐ **Zand Decongest Herbal Formula:** An herbal formula used to clear nasal passages and reduce swollen sinus membranes.
- ☐ **Nature's Way Nature's Cold Care:** An herbal formula that provides temporary relief of nasal congestion and upper respiratory cold symptoms.
- ☐ **Power Herbs Bronc-ease:** An herbal formula used as a natural cough suppressant, expectorant, and nasal decongestant.
- ☐ **Energy Medicine Sinus:** A homeopathic formulation used for relief of stuffy nasal sinuses.
- ☐ **Olbas Inhaler:** An inhalant used to clear blocked nasal passages.
- ☐ **Breezy Balms Warm Up Rub:** An aromatic warming salve that can be used as a chest rub.
- ☐ **Breh Respiratory Rescue:** A bath salt containing aromatic oils formulated especially to help tone mucous membranes.
- ☐ **Autumn Harp Comfrey Salve:** An herbal salve containing olive oil and wheat germ oil (rich in Vitamins A, D, and E), used to relieve the discomfort and speed the healing of soreness or chapping around the nose.
- ☐ **Hyland's Calendula Off. 1X Ointment:** A homeopathic salve used to speed the healing of soreness or chapping around the nose.

If you are suffering from congestion due to cold or flu-like symptoms, a few products are available that may bring you some relief. One is another Zand product called the Zand Decongest Herbal Formula. This 100 percent natural formula clears nasal passages and reduces swollen sinus membranes.[42] Chinese ephedra (ma huang) is the active ingredient in this product that contains ephedrine in its natural state. This botanical is combined with a synergistic blend of herbs (a Chinese formula that has been used for centuries) and nutritional supplements (zinc and bioflavonoids). The fact that this formula contains no antihistamines, which have a tendency to cause drowsiness, does not affect its ability to bring effective sinus relief.

Another fine product for nasal congestion, produced by Nature's Way, is Nature's Cold Care. This natural cold-care medicine also uses the natural pseudoephedrine from the Chinese ephedra plant. In addition to this active ingredient, each capsule contains Vitamin C, bioflavonoids, trace minerals, and carefully selected herbs and herbal extracts. Nature's Cold Care provides temporary relief of nasal congestion and other upper respiratory cold symptoms, without causing drowsiness. It also reduces swelling of nasal membranes and promotes nasal and sinus drainage.[43]

Power Herbs Bronc-ease, manufactured by Nature's Herbs, is a wonderful, natural cold-care product. As a natural cough suppressant, expectorant, and nasal decongestant, it works with your body to help relieve cough due to minor throat and bronchial irritation. It also loosens phlegm, rids the bronchial passageways of mucus, relieves irritated membranes in the respiratory passageways, and relieves the nasal congestion that may occur with the common cold.[44] The active ingredients include extracts of white pine bark, horehound, slippery elm, and pseudoephedrine as it occurs naturally in "certified potency" Chinese ephedra extract.

Energy Medicine Sinus is also a homeopathic product worth mentioning in relation to stuffiness in the nasal sinuses. This is a formulation of seven carefully derived remedies, which often help with sinus-type symptoms. I've personally seen good results with it.

The Penn Herb Company distributes a natural inhaler, conveniently pocket-sized for easy carrying (about the same dimensions as a lip-balm stick). The Olbas Inhaler, a product of Switzerland, is meant to be inserted in one nostril and its vapors inhaled while you hold the other nostril closed. Because it contains only menthol and oils of peppermint, cajuput (an Asian tree), and eucalyptus as the natural ingredients, there is no fear of habit-forming side effects. The Olbas Inhaler is quite effective in clearing nasal passages and in loosening the mucus accumulations that block sinus passages.

Many of us have experienced the relief and comfort a warming vapor rub can have when we have suffered from sinus or chest congestion. Most of the medications of this type are in a petroleum base. I can, however, recommend a fine, non-petroleum product available. Breezy Balms Warm Up Rub combines the essential oils of camphor, eucalyptus, thyme, cajuput, and wintergreen in a base of olive oil and beeswax. This formulation not only provides deep heating to the area of the skin where it is applied, but also releases aromatic vapors that help clear stuffy sinuses. Warm Up Rub is very comforting when applied to the chest, forehead, or sinuses. Homeopathic preparations are often rendered inactive when camphor is used, so you might not want to use this product in combination with a homeopathic remedy or formulation.

One other product worth mentioning is Breh Respiratory Rescue, which combines the extracts and oils of yarrow, rosemary, ginger, elder, eucalyptus, and tea tree with mineral-rich bath crystals to give you a specific bath salt formulation for respiratory problems. There is nothing like a hot bath when feeling "under the weather" and this bath salt adds an additional healing dimension. This formula is designed to help the body defend itself from sinus illnesses and viral invasions by eliminating toxins through perspiration while toning mucous membranes. Using the principles of immersion therapy, herbology, and aromatherapy, Breh officials advise us to use this product with warmer bath temperatures and without the use of soaps, which may alter the effect of the essential oils.

Immersion therapy refers to the ability of the skin to absorb substances into the body. For example, if you were to take slices of fresh garlic and place them on the soles of your feet, before long you would taste garlic on your breath. Similarly, by soaking in a bath containing herbs, the body can absorb the herbs. This method is often an effective way to give herbs to small children. Aromatherapy refers to a therapy that uses the ability of odors to alter moods and even body chemistry. Breh uses these methods in this and other products I will be mentioning.

A nasty side effect of having a sinus problem accompanied by a runny nose is the soreness that can develop around and within the nose due to chapping. Two products that may bring some relief for irritated skin around the nostrils are Autumn Harp Comfrey Salve and Hyland's Calendula Off. 1X Ointment. We will look at both of these products in more detail in Chapter 9.

One other sinus condition worth mentioning is sinusitis. Sinusitis is simply an inflammation and usually an infection of the membranes lining the sinuses, where interference of normal drainage has occurred.[45] Because proper drainage of the sinuses cannot take place, a perfect environment for bacterial growth is provided. It affects one or more of the eight sinus cavities in the heads of thirty to fifty million Americans. It is characterized by a painful condition often felt in the nose, forehead, eyes, and even the teeth, and a thick, greenish or yellowish discharge from the nose and down the back of the throat (postnasal drip). Most sinus conditions start to improve after about three days even though they may drag on for a week or so. Sinusitis, on the other hand, tends to get worse after two to three days and continues to worsen. Medical attention should be considered if this condition exists.[46]

Three factors contribute to this agonizing condition: allergies, environmental irritants, and structural abnormalities. Congestion from allergic reactions can block passage of mucus as can industrial pollutants, automobile exhausts, and tobacco smoke. Sometimes, the cartilage and bone wall that separates the passages in the nose may become crooked, usually as a result of an automobile accident, a sports injury, or a similar trauma. This condition, known as a deviated septum, can interfere with normal drainage of certain nasal cavities.

For some people, sinusitis can be a frequently occurring, extremely painful ailment. Some of the products mentioned under other headings in this chapter may offer some relief. Humidifying the air and drinking lots of fluids may help keep the mucus flowing, and avoiding dust, pollen, and pollution may also assist in preventing the problem. For some with structural abnormalities, correcting the deviation through surgery may be the only avenue of relief. Though this alternative may sound undesirable, it has been shown to be extremely effective and may outweigh the pain and misery of years of suffering.

Sore Throat and Coughs

A sore throat is usually one of the first signs that the body's defenses are at work against an aggressor threatening our health. The symptoms of pain and irritation in the throat are due to swollen lymph glands, where the remains of our white blood cells and enemy bacterial cells have accumulated after doing battle. Though supplements that strengthen our resistance should be our first line of defense, we also need to soothe the irritation of a sore throat. There are a few natural products available to ease this discomfort.

Some Natural Products Used for Sore Throats and Coughs:

- [ ] **Camocare Throat Spray/Gargle:** An herbal formulation used to soothe irritated throat tissue.
- [ ] **Naturade Expec:** An herbal syrup used to loosen mucus buildup and maintain free breathing in nasal passages.
- [ ] **Naturade Expec II:** An herbal syrup used to provide soothing temporary relief of dry hacking cough.
- [ ] **Naturade Expec III Throat Lozenges:** An herbal lozenge used to provide temporary relief of coughs, sore throat, and mouth dryness.
- [ ] **Kal LoZINCges:** A zinc-enriched lozenge used to soothe sore throats and bring some relief for cough sufferers.
- [ ] **Zand HerbaLozenge:** An herbal lozenge used to cool and soothe irritated throat tissues.
- [ ] **Zand HerbaLozenge Vitamin C Orange:** A Vitamin C-enriched throat lozenge used to soothe irritated throat tissue.
- [ ] **Power Herbs Bronc-ease:** An herbal formula used as a natural cough suppressant, expectorant, and nasal decongestant.
- [ ] **Breezy Balms Warm Up Rub:** An aromatic warming salve that can be used as a chest rub.

One product by Abkit, Inc., called Camocare Throat Spray/Gargle, comes with a handy attachment so you can spray it into your throat or, if you prefer, simple gargle it. Because the essential oil of the chamomile plant from which this spray is made has a low-water solubility, chamomile tea contains only 10 to 15 percent of the plant's oil content. Camocare has developed a method to produce a standardized herbal product containing a potent amount of the chamomile oils. The unique formulation of natural oils combined with soothing chamomile goes to work immediately to bring relief to irritated throat tissues.

The Naturade Company provides three noteworthy products for symptoms associated with cough and sore throat problems. Naturade Expec and Naturade Expec II are both herbal combination syrups. The Expec product is a pleasant-tasting formula, which, by its soothing action, helps loosen mucus buildup and maintain free breathing passages due to colds, flu, hay fever, and smog. It can also relieve minor sore throat pain caused by excess coughing. Expec II provides soothing temporary relief of dry hacking cough due to the common cold or inhaled irritants. This cough syrup contains such renowned natural ingredients as bee propolis, licorice root, echinacea, rose hips, lemon balm, slippery elm, mullein, and others. Expec can be used by children as young as three years old and Expec II can even be used by two-year-olds.

The third Naturade product is a sore throat lozenge in a base of natural herbs and bee propolis. Naturade Expec III Throat Lozenges provide temporary relief of coughs, sore throat, and mouth dryness, resulting from colds, flu, or smoking. This non-narcotic formula contains many of the herbs in the Expec syrups, has a very pleasant taste, and is free of sugar. It even contains pure chlorophyll as a natural breath freshener (bad breath often accompanies a sore throat).

Kal LoZINCges, mentioned earlier in this chapter, can also be used to soothe sore throats and bring some relief for cough sufferers. One of the ingredients, slippery elm, has been used since the time of the American Indians for its soothing effect on mucous membranes.[47] It also contains zinc and Vitamin C, two excellent supplements to aid our body's defenses.

Another product for throat irritation is the Zand HerbaLozenge, produced by Zand Herbal Formulas. The owners of this company set out to develop a throat lozenge without sugar. They felt that simple sugars metabolize "acidic" in the body and, in some individuals, this was a favorable environment for bacteria and virus to multiply. Not what one would want when suffering with sore throats, coughs, or congestion. While Dr. Zand was clinically testing a blend of Chinese and Western herbs renowned for their cooling and soothing properties, rice syrup was selected as the sweetener for the lozenge. The result is a mint-flavored, herbal-mentholated lozenge, containing added to their line with a Vitamin C-enriched lozenge, Zand HerbaLozenge Vitamin C Orange. Like the menthol cough drop, it is sweetened with only rice syrup.

If you are suffering from a recurrent cough, Power Herbs Bronc-ease by Nature's Herbs may bring some relief. This fine product was discussed in detail under the topic of sinus congestion. Also, the warming action of Breezy Balms Warm Up Rub may bring comfort and relief to chest conditions. Remember, because of the nullifying action that camphor can have on the effectiveness of homeopathics, Warm Up Rub should not be used in conjunction with homeopathic preparations.

Hay Fever and Allergies

Each year during the spring and fall, millions of Americans suffer from allergy symptoms like nasal blockage, hay fever, and upper respiratory discomforts. According to the National Institute of Health, 35 to 40 million people fall prey to hay fever, and 12 million people suffer from other allergies, unrelated to pollen. In the late 1970s, the National Center for Health Statistics found that about 1 in 5 Americans between the ages of 6 and 74 are allergic to something. I would imagine that that figure has increased somewhat since this survey, due to the increase of pollutants available in our foods and in the environment.

For those of you who suffer from sinus problems due to hay fever or allergies, the search for products that can reduce the discomfort of such attacks can be a timely concern. Eliminating an allergy itself can be an expensive and lengthy process, working with a medical allergy specialist as he or she tests your reaction to hundreds of different substances. Our sensitivity may be to a food such as wheat, corn, dairy products, or a list of other common edibles. We may react to a variety of airborne plant pollens or to the spores of molds that sometimes accumulate in our environment, often breeding in our air conditioner systems. Dog hairs, cat hairs, dust, pesticides on fruits and vegetables, chemicals in cleaning solutions, and many other substances can make up the almost endless list of substances we can react to. Unfortunately, individuals may have an allergic reaction to a number of different substances and may not be able to isolate themselves completely from many of these irritating elements.

For this reason, hay fever and allergy sufferers reach for medications to relieve the symptoms of swollen membranes, sinus pressure, and restricted breathing. To compound the problem, many of the pharmaceutical preparations found at the drug store contain many impure ingredients. Artificial coloring, preservatives, sugar, and such synthetic chemical additives as hydroxypropyl methylcellulose, croscarmellose sodium, polyethylene glycol, polysorbate 60, sorbitan monolaurate, cetylpyridinium chloride, and microcrystalline cellulose are a few of the questionable ingredients found in common allergy medications. But there is hope. There are manufacturers who are dedicated to providing the public with safe alternatives to relieve the suffering caused by substance sensitivity.

Some Natural Products Used for Hay Fever and Allergies:

- [ ] **Nature's Herbs Allerin:** A full-potency natural-source allergy medicine used for hay fever, allergies, and sinus problems.
- [ ] **Power Herbs Allerelief:** A natural-source nasal decongestant used for hay fever, allergies, and sinus problems.
- [ ] **Nature's Way Allerex:** A maximum-strength natural allergy medicine that provides temporary relief for hay fever, nasal congestion, and respiratory allergies.
- [ ] **Nature's Way Broncrin:** An herbal product used for the relief of respiratory symptoms due to bronchial asthma.
- [ ] **Bioforce Pollinosan:** A homeopathic formulation used to relieve the discomfort associated with allergies and hay fever.
- [ ] **Longevity Hayfever:** A homeopathic formulation used for relief of the symptoms of runny nose, sneezing, stuffiness, itching of the nose and throat, and itchy, watery eyes due to hay fever or other upper respiratory allergies.
- [ ] **bioAllers Allergy Relief: Animal Hair/Dander:** A homeopathic preparation used for relief of such symptoms as congestion, sneezing, asthmatic symptoms, and itching associated with animal allergies.
- [ ] **bioAllers Allergy Relief: Mold/Yeast/Dust:** A homeopathic preparation used for relief of such symptoms as sinus congestion, headaches, coughs, and sore throats associated with mold, yeast, and dust allergies.

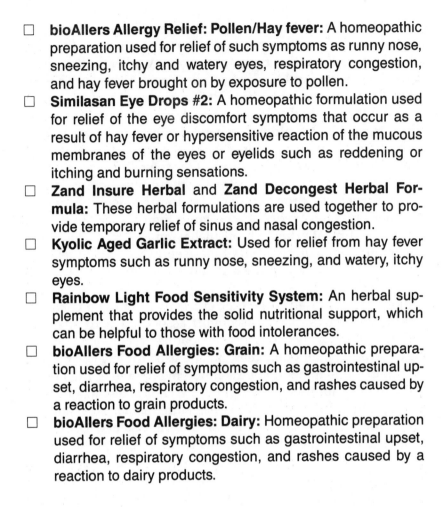

☐ **bioAllers Allergy Relief: Pollen/Hay fever:** A homeopathic preparation used for relief of such symptoms as runny nose, sneezing, itchy and watery eyes, respiratory congestion, and hay fever brought on by exposure to pollen.

☐ **Similasan Eye Drops #2:** A homeopathic formulation used for relief of the eye discomfort symptoms that occur as a result of hay fever or hypersensitive reaction of the mucous membranes of the eyes or eyelids such as reddening or itching and burning sensations.

☐ **Zand Insure Herbal** and **Zand Decongest Herbal Formula:** These herbal formulations are used together to provide temporary relief of sinus and nasal congestion.

☐ **Kyolic Aged Garlic Extract:** Used for relief from hay fever symptoms such as runny nose, sneezing, and watery, itchy eyes.

☐ **Rainbow Light Food Sensitivity System:** An herbal supplement that provides the solid nutritional support, which can be helpful to those with food intolerances.

☐ **bioAllers Food Allergies: Grain:** A homeopathic preparation used for relief of symptoms such as gastrointestinal upset, diarrhea, respiratory congestion, and rashes caused by a reaction to grain products.

☐ **bioAllers Food Allergies: Dairy:** Homeopathic preparation used for relief of symptoms such as gastrointestinal upset, diarrhea, respiratory congestion, and rashes caused by a reaction to dairy products.

One of these companies, Nature's Herbs, offers two excellent products to allergy sufferers. Allerin and Power Herbs Allerelief are both effective products for many victims of hay fever, allergies, and sinus problems. Both products help reduce swollen membranes and nasal passages, decongest sinus openings and passages, relieve sinus pressure, and can temporarily restore freer breathing through the nose.[48] Both are made without synthetic drugs, aspirin, or antihistamines (which cause drowsiness). Allerin is billed by Nature's Herbs as a full-potency, natural-source allergy medicine and Allerelief as a natural-source nasal decongestant. Both are very good products.

Another manufacturer providing natural allergy relief is Nature's Way. Their Allerex product is a maximum-strength natural allergy medicine that provides temporary relief for hay fever, nasal congestion, and respiratory allergies.[49] Allerex utilizes 60 milligrams of pseudoephedrine HCl, a natural ephedrine found in the Chinese ephedra plant. Again, because of the absence of antihistamines, this product can relieve symptoms associated with upper respiratory allergies without causing drowsiness.

Nature's Way also offers a product for the relief of respiratory symptoms due to bronchial asthma without causing the side effect of drowsiness. Broncrin is an all-natural bronchodilator that provides temporary relief of wheezing, tightness of chest, and shortness of breath due to bronchial asthma. Again, the active ingredient is ephedrine (from Chinese ephedra), which relieves the constricting of the bronchial tubes and allows air to flow more freely.[50]

Bioforce Pollinosan is another excellent product to consider when suffering from the discomfort associated with allergies and hay fever. Pollinosan is a homeopathic preparation consisting of seven different remedies that are used for hay fever, allergic rhinitis (inflammation of the lining membrane of the nose), and nervous rhinitis-type symptoms. In clinical tests conducted from spring to fall, 1980 by M. Wiesenaure, S. Haussler, and W. Gaus, favorable results of one of the ingredients, *Galphimia glauca* prompted the creation of this Swiss homeopathic medicine. In this clinical double-blind study involving patients who suffered from acute hay fever (pollinosis), the patients showed an average of 80 percent improvement in their symptoms, and many experienced total relief when they used the homeopathic form of this Central American plant.[51]

I have a business associate who swears by Pollinosan, claiming that of all the different natural products she has tried for her hay fever problems, this is the only one that brought her relief. Of course, we all have different biological make-ups, which enable different products to bring the results desired by different individuals, but this is definitely a product worth trying if you are looking for hay fever or allergy relief.

There are several homeopathic preparations on the market that can help with hay fever symptoms. Another one I prefer is Longevity Hayfever by Longevity Pure Medicine. This product can offer help with such symptoms as runny nose, sneezing, stuffiness, itching of the nose and throat, and itchy, watery eyes due to hay fever or other upper respiratory allergies.[52] It also comes in an easy-to-use container, which, due to the delicate nature of such homeopathic remedies, helps to prevent any contamination.

Natra-Bio produces a line of allergy products under the bioAllers trade name. These products are designed to help with allergy symptoms for specific allergic reactions. If you know just what causes your allergies, the best defense is to avoid the irritating substance, but, of course, that is not always easy to do. When you are not able to stop the causes, these fine homeopathic combinations can at least be used to help relieve the symptoms.

BioAllers Allergy Relief: Animal Hair/Dander, bioAllers Allergy Relief: Mold/Yeast/Dust, and bioAllers Allergy Relief: Pollen/Hayfever are available to combat the specific allergens as described by their product names. Allergy Relief: Animal Hair/Dander can provide relief of congestion, sneezing, asthmatic symptoms, and itching associated with animal allergies. Allergy Relief: Mold/Yeast/Dust may be of help with sinus congestion, headaches, coughs, and sore throats associated with mold, yeast, and dust allergies. And Allergy Relief: Pollen/Hayfever can bring relief of such symptoms as runny nose, sneezing, itchy and watery eyes, respiratory congestion, and hay fever brought on by exposure to pollen.[53] All three are worth experimenting with if you know the cause of your allergy discomfort.

Another condition that often accompanies hay fever is an itching and burning of the eyes. If you find yourself suffering from this problem, there is a product that can bring your eyes gentle soothing help. Similasan Eye Drops #2 is a preparation that can, according to homeopathic principles, give relief for hay fever-induced eye discomforts. This product will be discussed in more detail in Chapter 6.

Two other products worth mentioning here have already been written about in detail. Both products are produced by Zand: Zand Insure Herbal and Zand Decongest Herbal Formula. For temporary relief of sinus and nasal congestion, these products can be used together during the hay fever season.[54]

Research has been done on the effects of Kyolic Aged Garlic Extract on allergies, especially those created by airborne pollutants. (This product was covered at length in the section on immune function earlier in this chapter.) In *Garlic and Health*, Dr. Benjamin Lau describes several laboratory studies and individual case studies of the effects of Kyolic on heavy-metal contamination. Heavy metals are among the common air pollutants thought to be responsible for many allergic conditions. Some individuals have found relief from hay fever symptoms such as runny nose, sneezing, and watery, itchy eyes with the addition of Kyolic supplements to their diets.[55]

I'd like to mention a few more things specifically concerning food allergies. This is a problem that has become more and more widespread in recent years. Sensitivities to food substances can result in symptoms such as diarrhea, cramping, bloating, headaches, dizziness, postnasal drip, watery eyes, excessive congestion, anxiety, depression, and "a feeling of distraction." There is a great deal still to be learned about food sensitivities, but many natural food advocates believe that a breakdown in the digestive tract, as well as in the immune system, contribute to this problem.[56] A candida condition can also result in food sensitivities, but we will cover candida later in the book.

This breakdown occurs when we consume large levels of undigested fats and proteins, which are plentiful in our typical modern diets. The immune system, in response to these substances, dispatches agents including some known as IgE antibodies. When abnormally high levels of IgE antibodies settle in the tissues that make up the bowel walls, the tiny holes through which the nutrients pass tend to become enlarged. With these openings widened, larger, undigested proteins are allowed to pass through the intestinal wall into the bloodstream. At this point, the immune system attempts to neutralize these protein molecules with prostaglandins, leukotri-enes, and histamines. The result of these substances being constantly released into the bloodstream is the symptomology we call food sensitivities or food allergies.[57]

One product that has offered a solution to many sufferers of food intolerance is Rainbow Light Food Sensitivity System. The makers have formulated this supplement to restore integrity to both the digestive tract and the immune system. Rainbow Light Food Sensitivity System provides the solid nutritional support that can be immensely helpful to those with food intolerances.

This manufacturer has combined potent and nutritionally-balanced herbs with enzymes that help to digest foods completely. The enzymes work on all four of the food groups and function at all three stages of digestion. With these tools, the body can begin to rebuild the weaknesses that have occurred due to enzymatic and nutritional depletion.[58]

An additional benefit of Rainbow Light Food Sensitivity System is that if it does not perform to your expectations, you can return it with your sales receipt to the address on the bottle for a complete refund. I have deep respect for a company with this degree of confidence in their product.

If you know that grains or dairy products are the cause of your food sensitivity, two other products worth considering for food-related allergy symptoms are produced by the Natra-Bio Company under the bioAllers trade name. These homeopathic formulations, bioAllers Food Allergies: Grain, and bioAllers Food Allergies: Dairy, are designed to stimulate the body's natural defenses against symptoms from these specific food intolerances. Some symptoms caused by a reaction to grain or dairy products that these medications may help relieve include gastrointestinal upset, diarrhea, respiratory congestion, and rashes.[59] If you suffer from either grain or dairy intolerances, it might serve you well to keep the appropriate bioAllers formula on hand.

If you suspect that you may suffer from a food allergy, a very good self-help guide is *Hidden Food Allergies* by Dr. Stephen Astor. In this book, you will learn how to determine if you are one of the 33 percent of the population that suffers from this problem.[60] He maintains that the expensive tests of the allergy specialists, of which he is one, are only 20 percent accurate in determining your sensitivities to foods. Easy-to-follow guidelines help you determine for yourself if a food intolerance exists. His book also shows you how to pinpoint the specific food causing the problem, how to choose a qualified specialist to work with if needed, and how to treat your hidden allergies.

6

The Nervous System

The nervous system is a communication network that transmits information by electrical signals throughout the body. It accomplishes this function by using a vast chain of nerves that carry signals into and out of the central nervous system, namely the brain and spinal cord. The brain and, to a lesser extent, the spinal cord, interpret and process incoming signals and produce appropriate outgoing messages. The cerebrum, one of the higher centers of the brain, is generally considered to be responsible for thought processes and conscious activities. The nervous system, along with the endocrine system, controls and coordinates the workings of the brain. The endocrine organs influence the brain by secreting hormones that have an effect on many of the messages that are sent out by the brain.

Two kinds of cells make up the nervous system. The neurons (nerve cells) conduct and process electrical impulses between areas of the body. These cells perform the major work of the nervous system. Neurologia, the other type of cell, possess a special kind of connective tissue. They do not transmit impulses, but rather serve to support, repair, and perhaps nourish the neurons.[1]

Neurons conduct electrical impulses in a specific direction from one end to the other. Just as electrical wires are coated with an insulative material, so neurons have a nonconductive coating called myelin surrounding them; signals from one nerve do not interfere with signals from another. There are three types of neurons. Sensory neurons carry messages into the central nervous system and motor neurons transport messages out of the central nervous system. A third type of neuron, called an interneuron, transmits messages between sensory and motor neurons within the central nervous system.

The impulse signals themselves are electrochemical in nature, produced by the rapid in-and-out exchange of sodium and potassium ions. This process sweeps along the length of the neuron, from one end to the other. This impulse moves faster on larger, thicker nerve cells and varies from 0.5 meter per second for the smallest nerve fibers to 100 meters per second in the largest!

When one considers how many different kinds of messages are transmitted in order for a human body to function properly, the importance of the nervous system starts to become obvious. Each neuron is sensitive to only one type of stimulus. For example, one sensory neuron is needed in each area of the skin to send the message of each of the basic sensations of pain, touch, temperature, and pressure. In addition, a specific temperature-sensory neuron is needed for "cold," another for "heat," and still another for "very cold." Consider all the different functions of the digestive system and how many different signals are needed to accomplish the digestion of just one meal! How about the numerous movements of the hundreds of muscles throughout our body? I could go on and on. Suffice it to say, there is a real necessity to keep our nervous system healthy and functional. Through proper nutrition we can avoid and correct many symptoms associated with an unhealthy or imbalanced nervous condition.

Headaches

Whether headache pain is from an ordinary headache or from the more serious migraine type, it is always an unwelcome guest. Though the pain of a headache is experienced by the nervous system, the actual cause may be digestive-related. In many cases, fermentation occurs when our digestive system is not operating properly. This condition may be due to an unhealthy gastrointestinal tract or to the ingestion of poor foods or poor combinations of foods. Fermentation occurs in the digestive tract and leads to gas. Some of this gas is absorbed into the circulatory system where the blood transports it to different parts of the body. When these tiny bubbles of gas enter the very tiny capillaries in the head, the pressure they create can be felt as a headache. Poor digestion is not the only cause of headaches, but it is suspected to be the cause of many of these painful disturbances.

Tension is another major cause of headache pain. Of course, tension can affect our digestion as well. Then, poor digestion becomes an indirect cause of a headache. When we are under stress and experiencing tension, energy, which might be used in digestive processes, is not available for this function. The result again is incomplete digestion with gaseous by-products.

Some other causes of headaches, both occasional and the more severe migraines, include: allergies to foods and industrial or household chemicals, caffeine addiction, hypoglycemia (low blood sugar), food additives (especially MSG and nitrates), oral contraceptives or estrogen supplements, premenstrual hormonal imbalances, and poor functioning of many different organs of the body. Some people can even bring on a headache by sleeping with their heads under the covers. Dr. Gordon J. Gilbert wrote of this "turtle headache" in the *Journal of the American Medical Association* in 1972. He explained that sleeping in this manner can create a shortage of oxygen and a build-up of carbon dioxide, which, in turn, can cause you to wake up with a headache in the morning.[2]

A correspondence between the back of the neck and the forehead should be noted. It is here, in the rear of the brain, that our occipital lobes are located and the functions of sight are controlled. When we strain our eyes by reading in poor light or by concentrating on our work for an extended time, for example, we may develop a headache. When we become tense, our neck and shoulders tighten up. This constriction can resonate as pressure on the forehead. That's why a headache can often be relieved simply by massaging the back of the neck.

The very best "hands-on" method I have ever found to bring relief for headache pain combines a couple of polarity techniques. The first involves holding two points, one on each foot about three-quarter inches behind the base of the toes where the second and third toes (counting from the smallest) come together. You can usually find a very tender point here between the two tendons. For several minutes, hold both feet firmly in this place, with the thumbs on top and the middle fingers on the bottom. After you have finished with the feet, place your left palm flat across the forehead. Then place the right hand behind the head at the top of the neck. You will feel a ridge (the occipital ridge) at the base of the rear of the skull. Place your thumb and middle finger just under this ridge about one inch on either side of the spine and apply pressure in the direction of the forehead. Hold these contacts for 3–5 minutes and try to remain as relaxed as possible while doing so. Quite often these simple techniques will bring relief for headache sufferers.

There are also some effective natural products available for headache relief. Because, as mentioned before, digestive and stress-related problems may contribute to headache pain, some of the digestive aids and stress-relief products mentioned in their respective chapters might be worth considering if you are suffering from recurrent problems.

Some Natural Products Used for Headaches:

- [ ] **Power Herbs Willowprin:** A certified potency extract of white willow bark used for relief of some headache symptoms.
- [ ] **Yerba Prima Feverfew:** An herb that has earned a reputation as a remedy for the treatment and prevention of certain types of migraine headaches.
- [ ] **Yerba Prima Dong Quai:** An herb used for the relief of some tension headaches. (tablet)
- [ ] **Nature's Herbs Dong Quai:** An herb used for the relief of some tension headaches. (capsule)
- [ ] **Energy Medicine Headache:** A homeopathic formulation used for the relief of headaches that tend to be in one location.
- [ ] **Energy Medicine Headache/Neuralgia:** A homeopathic formulation used for the relief of headaches that move from place to place or are causing discomfort in more than one area of the head.

When I have a headache, the product I often get good results with is Power Herbs Willowprin by Nature's Herbs. Willowprin is a certified potency extract of white willow bark in a base of the same herb. White willow bark is the original source of salicin, the forerunner of aspirin, though weaker in activity. The Greeks, Egyptians, and American Indians used this herb to relieve pain of many types, not only headache, but also fever, gout, arthritis, sore muscles, and angina.[3] In 1853, researchers first produced acetylsalicylic acid (now known as aspirin) from salicylic acid, which in turn was made from the oxidation (the process of combining with oxygen) and hydrolysis (the addition of the elements of water) of salicin. Though salicin is found in small quantities in white willow bark, Willowprin contains enough salicin (at least 15 percent) to make it capable of providing relief for people with pain susceptible to aspirin-like compounds. At the same time, this product contains no aspirin, caffeine, preservatives, or synthetic drugs.

One well-researched herbal used for headache relief, especially migraines, is feverfew, a small flowering plant native to Europe. Feverfew has traditionally been used to relieve pain and reduce fever. Much of the research on this herb has been done by the London Migraine Clinic, Chelsea College. There in 1984, a double-blind study (meaning both groups did not know if they were given feverfew or a placebo) scientifically substantiated feverfew's effectiveness. In one survey, more than 70 percent of 270 migraine-headache sufferers who had eaten feverfew leaves for extended periods reported the herb had decreased the frequency or intensity of their attacks. Many of these subjects had failed to respond to orthodox medicine.[4]

A double-blind, placebo-controlled crossover study recently published in *The Lancet*, a highly respected British medical journal, has confirmed the beneficial activity of feverfew, as well. A placebo is a dummy pill that resembles the substance that is being tested, but is neutral in its effect. Seventy-two subjects were observed over a nine-month period. The first month, all were on a placebo. The next four months, half were on a placebo and half on feverfew. The last four months, the placebo group was put on feverfew and the other group was put on a placebo. Feverfew reduced the number of migraine attacks by 24 percent with a reduction of accompanying nausea and vomiting.[5] Although feverfew's pain-relief properties are evident, its effect on preventing migraines is still being studied. Research has shown that its effects may take from one week to three months to obtain the desired results against various types of migraine headaches.[6]

Yerba Prima Feverfew is an excellent feverfew supplement. In accordance with specifications outlined by doctors at the London Migraine Clinic, Yerba Prima's product is:

1. Made from the wild variety of feverfew (*Tanacetum parthenium*).
2. A freeze-dried product (to assure freshness and potency).
3. In the form of a 50-milligram tablet (typical dosage is 50 to 100 milligrams per day).

Feverfew has earned a deserved reputation as a remedy for treatment and prevention of certain types of migraine headaches, especially those that are relieved by applying warmth to the head.[7]

Dong quai, a Chinese herb, is another product worth mentioning for relief of headache pain. (The name is sometimes spelled tang kuei; its Latinized name is *Angelica sinesis*.) Dong quai is best known as a supplement for the female reproductive system and will be discussed in more detail under the subject devoted to female problems. However, another function this herb performs is the strengthening and relaxing of the muscles, and therefore it produces a calming effect on the nerves. As mentioned earlier, headaches are often associated with stress as well as tightness in the back of the neck. Dong quai, an antispasmodic herb,[8] tends to relax the muscles in the neck as well as other parts of the body. I have seen that two or three dong quai tablets taken when a headache problem occurs often brings relief of headache pain.

Yerba Prima Dong Quai is an excellent supplement of this wonderful herb. Each of its tablets contains 300 milligrams of concentrated dong quai root extract, standardized at 1 percent ligustilide (the active ingredient). Nature's Herbs also produces a good dong quai product. Nature's Herbs Dong Quai contains 100 percent pure high-quality dong quai in each capsule.

Two good homeopathic products may help the headache sufferer. Both are produced by Dolisos America Inc. and both are combinations of several remedies. Each of the remedies is designed to relieve specific types of headache symptoms. If your headache type conforms to a specific symptom relieved by one of the remedies in one of these combinations, relief can come so quickly that it may surprise you. And if your headache is not the right type for either of these combinations, as with other mild homeopathics, they will pass from your body with no ill effects.

The first combination, Energy Medicine Headache, is for headaches that tend to be in one location, such as the forehead. The other product is for headaches that move from place to place or are causing discomfort in more than one place, such as both the forehead and the back of the neck. Energy Medicine Headache/ Neuralgia is the combination remedy to try in this latter case. Between these two products, many common headaches can be remedied.

Stress and Eye Discomfort

Stress is one reason why so many of us feel in less than optimum health so much of the time. The complexities of modern life affect us on many levels, constantly overtaxing our physical and emotional capabilities. So many of us live in crowded cities with busy schedules, drive in heavy traffic, and are forever in the presence of air and noise pollution. All this puts a constant strain on our nerves. We may work long hours indoors with less than adequate exercise and often under stressful working conditions. Whether you work in an office environment or you are an active housewife dealing with the many details of keeping home and family together and comfortable, nervous tension and a tired body are most likely familiar to you.

The accumulated effects of the fast pace of living, traffic, air and noise pollution, busy schedules and the complicated jobs and activities that go with them, not to mention complex emotional relationships, all take their toll on our overall health. Stress is our body's natural response to danger. It releases hormones that aid in our responding to potential harm. This response, sometimes nicknamed the "fight or flight" response, has allowed us to evolve over millions of years. Until only recently in man's history, we had to overcome tremendous obstacles on a daily basis just to stay alive. Normally, we no longer need to respond physically to danger on such a steady basis, so these hormones are not eliminated as they once were. Left to build up in the body, the hormones create toxins that can weaken the systems of the body, causing a condition we've come to know as stress.

What can we do to remain healthy and balanced when we constantly have to deal with the added pressures that accompany modern lifestyles? B vitamins are essential nutrients for the nerves and can often help ease nervous tension. Taking a B-

Complex vitamin supplement is always a good idea when we are exposed to stressful situations. Since 1947, researchers have been studying herbs that have particular benefits in boosting overall health in the midst of stress.[9] These botanicals are classified as adaptogens, and have been shown to increase the human body's ability to adapt to abnormal environmental factors, both physical and psychological.

Some Natural Products Used to Combat Stress:

- ☐ **Yerba Prima Adaptoplex:** A combination of adaptogenic herbs used to provide the nutritional support needed to cope with stress.
- ☐ **Bach Rescue Remedy:** A flower remedy used to balance mental energies experienced as stress, irritability, loss of control, etc.
- ☐ **Hyland's Calms:** A homeopathic formulation used to relieve simple nervous tension and sleeplessness.
- ☐ **Kyolic Aged Garlic Extract:** Research shows garlic supplements provide stress-relieving benefits.
- ☐ **Breh Calm Seas:** A bath salt containing extracts and oils of a variety of sedative and relaxing herbs.
- ☐ **Living Source Complete B-Complex Nutrient System:** An excellent B-Complex vitamin supplement made with low-potency "food-bound" nutrients.
- ☐ **Similasan Eye Drops #1:** A homeopathic formulation used for relief of the eye-discomfort symptoms including red, fatigued, strained eyes due to smog, watery eyes with a sensation of grittiness, or hypersensitivity to light with inflammation of the eyelids.
- ☐ **Similasan Eye Drops #2:** A homeopathic formulation used for relief of the eye-discomfort symptoms that occur as a result of hay fever or hypersensitive reaction of the mucous membranes of the eyes or eyelids such as reddening or itching and burning sensations.

The finest adaptogen product I have found is Yerba Prima's Adaptoplex, a synergistic formula of four of the most powerful and balanced adaptogenic herbs. One of these ingredients, Siberian ginseng (*Eleuthrococcus* root), has been described by researchers as "a universal helping herb that increases man's adaptive capabilities."[10] It has a long history of use in China, is widely used in Russia, and has been studied in more than 1,000 research projects. Another ingredient, schizandra berry extract, has also been used for thousands of years in China and works as a powerful antioxidant to counteract the effects of toxins. Shiitake mushroom mycelia are also added to provide nutrients shown to help the body fight fatigue. And finally, American ginseng (*Panax quinquefolium*) is included for its deep, energy-building qualities. The American Indians used ginseng for its ability to build endurance without overstimulation.[11]

Adaptoplex works nutritionally to normalize the body's stress response and to prevent the build-up of dangerous toxins. This helps eliminate the fatigue and weakening that comes with overstimulation. It also helps protect and strengthen the body's natural resistance, and aids cellular energy production during periods of physical or emotional stress. If stress is wearing on you, I suggest you experiment with Adaptoplex. The benefits, from my experience, are quite often noticeable. I take two tablets in the morning when I see an intense workday approaching. When I don't foresee it, I take a couple to relieve the effects of stress.

Bach Rescue Remedy is also an excellent product to have on hand for use when stress is a factor in one's life. Impatiens, one of the five floral ingredients, is specifically for extreme mental stress and irritability, which causes muscle tension and pain.[12] Additional ingredients help with some of the other emotional conditions that affect us when we are exposed to stressful situations. Other floral ingredients include: rock rose (for terror, panic, fear), clematis (for faintness, coma, unconsciousness), cherry plum (for hysteria, loss of control, suicidal impulses), and star-of-Bethlehem (for shock, trauma). These five flowers, which are prepared in a special way, do not act directly upon a physical symptom, but rather on the condition of the mind that is generally present during emergencies or upsetting situations.[13]

Hyland's Calms is a homeopathic preparation, which has provided relief for many sufferers of simple nervous tension and sleeplessness. Calms is a formulation of four different remedies noted for their calming influences. Considered completely safe for regular use and non habit-forming, the manufacturer of this product claims it to be a "legal" daytime sedative. This is due to the fact that, after taking the product, it is safe to drive a car without any fear of drowsiness. This product is also considered safe for use with nervous children.[14]

There has also been research done in Japan, as well as here in America, showing the beneficial effects of garlic supplements in relieving stress. Dr. Benjamin Lau, M.D., Ph.D., in his book *Garlic and Health* describes several of these studies. In one involving over 1000 patients in seven university-teaching hospitals in Japan, 50 to 80 percent of the patients who ate Kyolic Aged Garlic Extract suffered less fatigue, depression, and anxiety than those who had taken no garlic supplements.[15] So, you may want to consider Kyolic (which we spoke about in detail when discussing the immune system in Chapter 5) as an addition to your diet if stress is influencing your life.

Another product that may be helpful in reducing the effects of stress is a specialized bath salt by the Breh Company. Breh Calm Seas is a formulation containing extracts and oils of a variety of sedative and relaxing herbs combined with unrefined, mineral-rich sea crystals. Through the principles of immersion therapy, herbology, and aromatherapy, this formula is designed to calm your mind and help take you inside yourself, thereby aiding you in focusing your energy.

Since B vitamins are so very important to the proper functioning of the nervous system, when stress is an imposition on your life, you may want to consider adding a good B-complex supplement to your diet. The best, in my opinion, is Living Source Complete B-Complex Nutrient System by Rainbow Light Nutritional Systems. These nutrients are produced by feeding synthetic vitamins to yeasts and then harvesting the yeast and thus obtaining a more naturally occurring form of the vitamins. The Grow Company developed this process and now produces these Food Grown or Grow Renatured nutrients for Rainbow Light. Though it may seem that a low-potency vitamin source would be inferior to the commonly used higher-dosage synthetic formulas, over fifty studies on absorption and retention of both types of vitamin sources prove just the opposite.[16]

In one such study done by Joe A. Vinson, Ph.D., associate professor of analytical chemistry at the University of Scranton, ten groups of rats were fed a Vitamin B-12-deficient diet for two weeks. After this period, the rats were given either synthetic Vitamin B-12 or Grow Renatured B-12 (used in Living Source products) in three different dosage levels. The results of the experiment showed a 256 percent better bio-availability of B-12 in the blood serum and a 159 percent better bio-availability of B-12 in the liver in the groups using the Grow Renatured B-12. Not only do I feel that Living Source Complete B-Complex Nutrient System is the best B-complex available, so does Rainbow Light, which backs its product with a full refund if you are not completely satisfied with its results.

Most people are not aware that stress can cause drying of the eyes. This may cause your eyes to burn and itch. Many other conditions responsible for eye discomfort, such as eyestrain from working at a computer, reading, driving at night, or not wearing an updated eyeglass prescription, are but a few factors that might lead one to use an eyecare product. Hay fever symptoms, rubbing the eyes, or the entry of some foreign substance into the eye can also cause discomfort. Fortunately, there are some natural eye drops available that are capable of bringing relief for inflammations and allergies.

Similasan AG of Switzerland produces two homeopathic drops for various eye discomforts. Similasan Eye Drops #1 are suggested if the symptoms include red, fatigued, strained eyes due to smog; watery eyes with a sensation of grittiness; or hypersensitivity to light with inflammation of the eyelids.[17] It is a calming, soothing, anti-inflammatory eye drop. Similasan Eye Drops #2 are used if the symptoms are a result of hay fever or there is a hypersensitive reaction of the eyes or eyelids such as reddening or itching and burning sensations of the eyes.[18]

With these two wonderful remedies on hand, you can be prepared to deal with many common eye complaints. Both products can be used by hard and soft contact lens wearers, are non-toxic, do not cause side effects, and are safe and effective for both adults and children.[19] Remember that these are sensitive homeopathic preparations and should be given the same care as oral remedies to preserve their delicate action as well as to protect your eyes. In other words, be careful not to contaminate the dropper opening with your fingers or use the drops at the same time as other foods and medicines.

If you are exposed to stress-producing conditions either on a daily basis or on occasion, there are several things that you can do.

First, give your body the nutritional support it needs with a good diet of healthful, unprocessed foods. Exercise is a natural way to release stress, so a regular exercise program can definitely be of benefit. Endorphins released during exercise help to relieve pent-up tensions. Give your body a chance to recuperate from the effects of stress with relaxation periods during the day, plenty of regular sleep at night, and other activities that offer relaxation such as a good massage or a hot tub or bath. And try some of the products mentioned here because they can often be of nutritional assistance in helping us cope with the stress in our lives.

Jet Lag, Minor Shock, and Travel Sickness

There are many different ways that shock can affect our systems. In more serious situations, it can be a life-threatening occurrence. In the event of a critical accident, a victim's state of shock must be treated quickly to avoid fatal problems, such as those caused by lack of oxygen to the brain. Standard first-aid procedures are to elevate the feet and keep the person warm. This helps to replenish blood supply to the brain cells because blood drains from the head when a person goes into shock. In less serious conditions, mild symptoms occur such as extreme fatigue. This is what happens when our body is exposed to several hours at high altitudes in the pressurized cabin of an airplane (jet lag). The exposure to radiation and ozone at higher altitudes also contributes to jet lag.[20] The rapid changing of time zones may also add distress to the natural rhythms that regulate body functions. All of these factors of jet travel disrupt the body's cellular harmony, creating an excess of toxic chemical molecules called free radicals. Free radicals are highly reactive molecules with an unpaired electron in their structure. When one undergoes a surgical operation, a shock to the system also occurs, making recovery period necessary. Whatever the cause or extent of the shock we might encounter, there are several natural products available, which can help our bodies adapt.

Some Natural Products Used for Jet Lag, Minor Shock, and Travel Sickness:

☐ **Yerba Prima Adaptoplex:** An adaptogenic herbal combination used to reduce the stressful effects of jet lag.

☐ **Hyland's Arnica 30X:** A homeopathic preparation used to relieve the symptoms of jet lag and minor shocks to the system.

☐ **Bach Rescue Remedy:** A flower remedy used to help relieve the emotional impact of shocking occurrences.

☐ **Power Herbs Travel-Ease:** An herbal formula that contains ginger root and acts on both the nervous and digestive systems to prevent the nausea and vomiting associated with motion sickness.

Yerba Prima's Adaptoplex is the first product I'd like to mention. (It was discussed in detail under the topic of stress). Because of the similarities between stress and minor shock, this product often helps with this condition as well. I use it to combat the effects of jet lag whenever I fly long distances. A couple of tablets before and after a flight are enough to keep me from experiencing any jet-lag symptoms on a three to five hour flight. Longer flights may need additional doses.

Two other products are worth your attention. A homeopathic preparation long known for its role in the relief of the stress associated with shocking occurrences is Hyland's Arnica 30X. Arnica is a preparation made from a plant found in the meadows or mountains of Europe and commonly known as the mountain arnica or leopard's-bane. Arnica can also be taken in a series of doses during a flight to combat jet lag and also after more serious shocks to the system.

Bach Rescue Remedy can also help relieve the emotional impact of shocking occurrences such as those stemming from an accident or injury or the loss of someone close. This product, mentioned earlier, helps to balance the emotions associated with traumatic conditions by lessening the effect of minor shock and by easing fear, panic, and pain. It has been used successfully to alleviate the distress of burns, hysteria, headaches, accidents, terror, birth, surgery, asthma, and everyday stresses in humans and can calm injured animals as well.[21] Of course, any time a person is suffering from a serious case of shock, medical attention should be sought immediately.

Since we are talking about jet lag, a condition brought about by traveling in our modern world, let me mention another type of traveling ailment suffered even before the advent of the commercial airliner. Travel or motion sickness is quite commonly experienced by many who travel by boat, automobile, or airplane. For those who suffer from motion sickness, even travel for pleasant reasons can be a very uncomfortable ordeal. Fortunately, there are some fine natural products available to help diminish this problem.

One is Power Herbs Travel-Ease. Motion sickness starts in both the gastrointestinal tract and the nervous system. The main ingredient in this product is powdered ginger root. Tests show that ginger root, especially in its powdered form, is effective in preventing motion sickness. In addition, studies show that ginger root acts on both the nervous and digestive systems to prevent nausea and vomiting, without causing the drowsiness found in pharmaceutical medicines.[22] If you experience a problem with motion sickness, Travel-Ease may help in preventing and treating the miserable symptoms associated with it.

Insomnia

Difficulty with sleeping can be an annoying problem, especially during periods of stress. Although insomnia is not well understood, most scientists agree that it is often a symptom of emotional stress, anxiety, or pain. When we do not get the quality of sleep we require, it can affect the strength of other systems of the body, which may lead to a susceptibility to illness.

Though Valium and other tranquilizers are generally prescribed for "nerves," many physicians also suggest them for insomnia. It is disturbing that the drug Valium is the most prescribed drug in the United States today when perfectly safe and effective natural products are readily available.[23] Over-the-counter sleeping pills can also lead to dependency and other harmful side effects. Fortunately, there are some natural alternatives to these more drastic medications. Please be cautioned, however, that the need to use a sleep inducer on a regular basis, whether it be a safe natural product or not, may signal a nutritional deficiency or the existence of a potentially serious illness.

Who knows how many people from how many cultures and for how many centuries have relied on warm milk to help induce sleep when they experienced trouble drifting off at night. Warm milk contains a bit of the amino acid tryptophan. Did you ever notice how sleepy you get after a Thanksgiving dinner? Turkey is also high in tryptophan. Dr. Julius Segal did research giving tryptophan to volunteers in sleep experiments at the National Institute of Mental Health. He found that they fell asleep with unusual speed, awoke less during the night, and spent more time than usual in the deep phases of sleep.[24] Most of the major natural vitamin companies produce an L-tryptophan supplement. The letter L used in front of the name means the amino acid is in the same natural form as in living plant or animal tissue. The L-forms of amino acids are considered more compatible with human biochemistry.

Unfortunately, at the time of this writing, there has been a temporary ban placed on all products containing added L-tryptophan. It seems that a rare blood disorder, eosinophilia myalgia syndrome, which elevates the white blood cell count, has been associated with the use of this supplement. Due to this recall by the FDA, L-tryptophan products have been removed from the shelves. Virtually all the cases in this investigation have been traced to a single Japanese supplier, Showa Denko, and a contaminated batch is suspected. Hopefully, this supplement, which has been used safely for years by millions of health-conscious individuals, will again become available for general use. But, fortunately, there are other natural sleep-inducing alternatives available to us.

Some Natural Products Used for Insomnia:

☐ **Yerba Prima Chamomile:** A good, calming herb that is used to help induce sleep.

☐ **Yerba Prima Valerian Root:** A sedative herb. It is helpful when taken shortly before bedtime to bring on sleep. Generally does not produce early morning drowsiness.

☐ **Nature's Way Naturest:** An herbal formulation that is used as a natural nighttime sleep aid.

☐ **Boiron Borneman Nervousness/Insomnia:** A homeopathic formulation used to provide relief of sleeplessness
and simple nervous tension.

☐ **Hyland's Calms:** A homeopathic formulation used to provide relief of sleeplessness and simple nervous tension.

There are several reputable herbs noted for their sedative
properties. A few you may be familiar with are chamomile,
hops (ever get sleepy after a beer?), basil, violet leaves, catnip,
passion flower, lemon verbena, and valerian root. A tea made
from a good sample of one or a combination of these herbs can
often help induce sleep. Yerba Prima Chamomile is a good
calming supplement that may help if you have problems falling
asleep. We learned about this product when we dealt with
indigestion.

Valerian root has a long history of use as a calming herb. It is
especially helpful when taken shortly before bedtime to bring
on sleep and generally does not result in early morning drowsiness. A number of valerian species are found in North America,
Asia, and Europe, but only *Valeriana officinalis* has been researched extensively. Evidence shows that in humans, this species
of valerian root is a strong sedative and also has a tendency to increase concentration and energy.[25] Studies have shown that a large
variety of nutrients contributes to its activity and that these can
vary from plant to plant.[26] These compounds found in the root,
called valepotriates, are the active constituents, and infiltrate the
brain tissue, blood cells, and the central nervous system, where
they produce a strong sedative effect on the entire body.[27] One of
the more important constituents is valerenic acid. Yerba Prima Valerian Root extract is a standardized product in tablet form, containing 0.5 percent valerenic acid. Besides being a very fine product, it is an easy way to ingest this herb, which tends to have an
unpleasant taste when taken as a tea.

Nature's Way Naturest is another excellent product to help induce sleep when it fails to come easily. Naturest is a natural nighttime sleep-aid that helps you to fall asleep easily. This product includes a standardized form of valerenic acid from valerian as well
as other sedative herbs. Its ingredients include catnip herb extract,
German chamomile flowers extract, hops flowers extract, and Ro-

man chamomile flowers extract. Taken in a capsule form, this, too, is a very effective product to help you avoid sleepless nights.

Two excellent homeopathic preparations exist for symptoms of insomnia and simple nervous tension. Each formulation is made up of a different combination of individual remedies, so, if one does not give you the results you desire, the other may. One of these, which consists of four individual remedies, is Boiron Borneman Nervousness/Insomnia. This product may help provide a gentle night's rest when sleep does not come easily. Hyland's Calms is another homeopathic formulation also known to help with sleeplessness. As with the Boiron product, this gentle non-prescription sedative consists of four homeopathic plant remedies, and is considered safe for children's use. It has provided relief for many sufferers of sleeplessness and simple nervous tension.[28]

There are a few other things I would like to mention regarding insomnia. Exercise, although not immediately before bed, may help to relax you enough to help you sleep at night. Also nighttime is not necessarily the only time to get our sleep. An afternoon nap, 20–90 minutes long, can not only add to the sleep you get, but can also help you sleep better at night. Dr. Philip M. Tiller, Jr., of the Louisiana State University School of Medicine, found this to be true when he conducted an experiment with several hundred women who complained of being run down, tired, and nervous. He had them take a one- or two-hour nap each afternoon. He determined that naps actually helped the women get a better night's sleep.[29] If you find it difficult to fall asleep, lie still and take slow deep breaths. It will help you to relax and let go of anxiety and tension.

Memory and Senility

As we age, we often tend to lose our mental edge. Our mental alertness and our concentration lose their sharpness and we sometimes forget many of the details of our daily life. Often this is caused by a degeneration of the delivery system responsible for supplying nutrients to these areas of the brain. Nerves do not rebuild themselves the same way skin cells or tissue cells do. This is particularly true of brain cells, which, after the age of seven, do not reproduce at all. If you lose a brain cell you lose it for good and, unfortunately, these cells are so sensitive in their need for oxygen, that only a few minutes without it can cause brain cell death.

Oxygen can also have a detrimental effect on us. Just as iron breaks down when it oxidizes (or rusts), when brain tissue oxidizes, brain cells break down and are destroyed. Damaging forms of oxygen called free radicals cause the breakdown of tissues in the body. Free radicals are highly reactive substances that come from external and internal sources such as stress, environmental pollution, and the by-products of certain heated cooking oils. They are a direct result of the chemical, physical, emotional, and infectious stresses we encounter.[30] They initiate chain reactions that can destroy the integrity of the body's cells. One way they destroy cells is by attaching themselves to and breaking down the proteins that make up the protective sheaths that surround the nerve cells.[31]

Another problem associated with aging is the slowing down of the circulatory system. This is due to the accumulation of cholesterol deposits on the walls of the blood vessels, making the passageways narrower. This, along with the clumping of red blood cells, slows the rate of the blood flow to the brain. Decreased circulation to the brain can affect it by starving it of needed oxygen and nutrients. Fortunately, there is a wonderful plant with a rich history to help bring renewed nourishment to our brain tissues.

Some Natural Products Used for Memory and Senility:

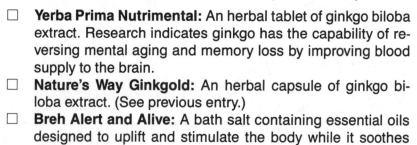

- ☐ **Yerba Prima Nutrimental:** An herbal tablet of ginkgo biloba extract. Research indicates ginkgo has the capability of reversing mental aging and memory loss by improving blood supply to the brain.
- ☐ **Nature's Way Ginkgold:** An herbal capsule of ginkgo biloba extract. (See previous entry.)
- ☐ **Breh Alert and Alive:** A bath salt containing essential oils designed to uplift and stimulate the body while it soothes the nerves.

Ginkgo biloba, also known as the maidenhair tree, is one of the oldest living species of trees. Its existence can be traced back over 200 million years, before the Ice Age. It is thought to be native to Northern China, and was cultivated in monasteries there as a sacred tree. This practice helped save the ginkgo from extinction when widespread deforestation practically eliminated the wild ginkgos.

Though the Chinese have used the ginkgo leaf in herbal preparations for thousands of years, modern Western scientists have provided documentation through hundreds of clinical studies showing the nutritional qualities of this botanical. Ginkgo is currently one of the best-selling herbs in Europe and Japan and is becoming more and more well known in other areas of the world.

Studies show ginkgo biloba extract helps to dilate blood vessels. This favors blood delivery to the tissues and allows for better elimination of wastes. The herb also helps to keep blood cells from sticking together causing clumps. In addition, ginkgo extract is an excellent free-radical scavenger, which helps slow the aging process and aids in the maintenance of healthy cells, especially in the area of the brain.[32] Ginkgo contains a specific combination of flavonoids and bioflavonoids (substances that increase the therapeutic effects of vitamins), which help penetrate areas that other nutrients have difficulty reaching. Except for occasional reports of headaches when taken for prolonged periods, ginkgo biloba has been shown to be without side effects, non-toxic, and to have no known interactions with other supplements.[33]

Current pharmaceutical research has been unable to uncover a drug that can efficiently and safely reverse mental aging. Hydergine-k (dihydroergotoxine) is the drug that is presently used, but it is not very effective and can be extremely toxic. Because of this, most physicians are hesitant to use it and feel helpless when confronted with patients suffering from senility. Ginkgo extract, on the other hand, appears to be extremely effective in such cases, as it works particularly well to reverse the aging process of the brain.[34] Dr. Vorberg of Munich, West Germany, achieved significant results in 1981, when he gave ginkgo extract to 112 patients aged 55 to 94, all suffering from chronic cerebral insufficiency. He was able to alleviate the following symptoms: vertigo, headache, tinnitus (ringing in the ears), short-term memory loss, vigilance (alertly watchful of danger), and mood disturbance. Vorberg's results have been substantiated in numerous other studies as well.[35]

Of the several quality botanical preparations manufactured that produce a ginkgo supplement, I prefer Yerba Prima Nutrimental and Nature's Way Ginkgold.

Nutrimental is a standardized product, guaranteed to contain the same amount of active ingredients used in research studies. This product is not only for the elderly. I'm in my early forties and can really feel a difference when my mind feels a little cloudy, for one reason or another, and I take Nutrimental. The clarity and concentration that replaces that cloudiness is a welcome experience. It may take several days or even longer to notice the effects, so be patient. I often hear people who take this herb comment on how clear and focussed it makes them feel. I also know of improvement in cases of senility when Nutrimental is taken regularly for several months. I'm sure this product can be a welcome supplement for the student after a late night of partying. It is definitely a good supplement to keep around the house for use when one feels the need.

Nature's Way Ginkgold is also an excellent ginkgo supplement that is prepared by one of Europe's leading companies in the field of natural research, Willmar Schwabe GmbH & Co. Each capsule contains 40 milligrams of ginkgo biloba in a neutral base of natural carbohydrate complex. Each extraction is carefully assayed and standardized as well, to assure consistent and dependable quality. From my personal experience, the Ginkgold product is another excellent source of the ginkgo herb.

Breh Alert and Alive is one other product to consider when you want to stimulate clarity and concentration. This synergistic combination of herbal extracts and oils is designed to uplift and stimulate the body while soothing the nerves. It is a tonic for the internal organs as well and is as easy to use as soaking in a hot bath with the bath crystals dissolved in it. Note, however, that using soap with this bath salt formula may detract from its effectiveness.

7

The Circulatory System

The circulatory system is the transportation network of the body. It provides a connection between the organs and each individual cell, either directly or indirectly. Via the circulatory system, each cell, no matter where in the body it is located, has fairly rapid access to the lungs for oxygen (or for the elimination of carbon dioxide), to the digestive tract for essential nutrients, and to the kidneys for elimination of cellular wastes. It also performs two other important functions. The endocrine system produces hormones that regulate bodily processes and the circulatory system transports these hormones to their site of action. In addition, the circulatory system transports antibodies and specialized bacteria-fighting white blood cells to areas where infection has occurred. Without this extensive transportation network, our other organ systems would be unable to function.

The circulatory system is made up of the blood, the heart, the blood vessels, and the capillaries. Blood is composed of several constituents that help to perform the various functions described in the previous paragraph. To go into detail describing the different cells and other substances that make up our blood and all the functions each performs would be quite lengthy and does not seem necessary in this text. It is sufficient to say that the blood carries out all these functions through various chemical reactions and physiological mechanisms. Meanwhile, the structures of the circulatory system allow the blood to move to all the regions of the body. The vessels and capillaries serve as channels to direct the blood through the body, and the heart acts as a sophisticated pump to keep the blood flowing.

There are three types of blood vessels: the arteries, the capillaries, and the veins. The arteries carry oxygenated blood away from the heart and lungs to other regions of the body. They are made up of smooth muscle and elastic tissue. The term "capillary" is derived from the Latin word for hair, indicative of their thinness. In reality, a capillary is several times thinner than a human hair. They are so numerous that if the capillaries from an adult human were laid end to end, they would circle the Earth two and a half times![1] The walls of capillaries are only one cell thick and, in most cases, blood cells pass through in single file. The capillaries allow the blood to maintain contact with the individual tissue cells for the exchange of oxygen, nutrients, and other substances. The third type of blood vessels are the veins, which carry the blood back to the heart and the lungs. They are less muscular and thinner than the arteries, and contain tiny valves along their length to prevent backflow when the blood pressure changes. Together, these three blood vessel types form the network that carries the blood to every tissue and cell in the body.

The heart is a four-chambered muscular organ that serves as a pump to circulate the blood throughout the body. It beats 2.5 billion times in the average lifetime, pumping approximately 1,750 gallons of blood daily.[2] The two upper chambers are called the atria and the lower chambers are called ventricles. The right atrium receives blood from all parts of the body and pumps it into the right ventricle below it. The right ventricle then pumps the blood towards the lungs where carbon dioxide is released and fresh oxygen is picked up. The blood returns to the left atrium where it is pumped into the left ventricle below. The left ventricle is the most muscular chamber of the heart, for it has to pump the oxygenated blood to all parts of the body except the lungs. Electrical impulses stimulate the chambers of the heart to pump in a seemingly perfect rhythm, producing the characteristic heart sounds. In the wall of the right atrium is the sinoatrial node, also called the pacemaker, which sets the rhythm of electrochemical impulses. In times of exertion, the heart pumps faster to supply needed oxygen to the muscles of the body.

The circulatory system works intricately with the other systems and organs of the body to keep the entire body nourished and synchronized. We often take our heart and other circulatory structures for granted, but their health is essential to our overall well-being. Knowing a little about good nutrition for the circulatory system can extend the life of these structures and, ultimately, the life of our bodies.

Heart Disease and Nutrition

The heart is one of the hardest-working organs of the body. Yet, as long as it functions properly, we usually give it little attention. By the ages of 16 to 20 years, over half of the American population show signs of hardening of the arteries. It is estimated that over 10 million people in the U.S. suffer from coronary heart disease and that this disease is responsible for over 1 million deaths yearly. Symptoms of heart dysfunction may include chest pain, fatigue with exertion, frequent coughing, increased anxiety, swelling in the lower legs, restlessness, paleness, and irregular heartbeat.[3]

There are numerous dietary practices that scientific research has shown contribute to diseases of the heart and circulatory system. Nicotine adds to the fatty buildup on artery walls causing decreased blood flow and, therefore, increased risk of heart disease. Deaths in general from coronary heart disease are 70 percent higher in smokers than in nonsmokers. A high caffeine intake can also increase one's susceptibility to heart attacks. A person who drinks six cups of coffee a day can raise the risk of heart disease by 120 percent![4]

A diet high in sugar can cause hardening of the arteries, as well. When a diet is high in refined carbohydrates such as white sugar or white flour, it can cause the liver to over-produce cholesterol. Because digestion of meat is not an easy task, a diet high in protein (over 15 percent by weight of total food intake) forces the heart to work 30 percent harder. Over an extended period, this can strain the heart. Evidence also suggests that excess protein increases cholesterol levels and subsequent hardening of the arteries. It is interesting to note that Seventh-Day Adventists, vegetarians all, suffer 84 percent less coronary heart disease than the general population. This group of people is known to abstain from tobacco, alcohol, caffeine, and meat.[5]

Stress is another factor contributing to problems of the cardiovascular system. We have already covered this topic in another area of the book. We know that stress interferes with our ability to properly digest and utilize the foods we eat, thereby costing us needed nutrition. I've also mentioned that exercise and other measures can help reduce the stress in our lives. It is not only possible for your blood pressure to rise under stressful conditions, it can also rise simply by thinking about a situation that has caused you stress.

Blood pressure is the pressure exerted by the blood as it flows through the circulatory system. If the heart beats faster and/or harder, or the arteries become narrower or lose their flexibility, blood pressure goes up. High blood pressure is an indication that the heart is working too hard to pump the blood throughout the body. Hypertension (high blood pressure) is sometimes referred to as the "silent killer" because in most cases you don't feel anything until some damage is done. It is estimated that one in four Americans (about 57 million individuals) has hypertension, whether they know it or not.[6] It is important to have your blood pressure tested at regular intervals: this condition can increase your risk of more serious complications.

Obesity may lead to heart disease. Overeating to the point of being overweight is extremely common in our society. Approximately 25 percent of men and women in America, between the ages of 20 and 74, are clinically obese, in other words 20 percent above their normal weight. Fifteen percent of children and 20 percent of teens are overweight as well.[7] It seems that obesity is virtually epidemic in this country. This is especially disconcerting considering the strain that carrying around excess weight can have on the heart.

It is interesting how common the knowledge is to anyone who has ever dieted that fats are something to steer clear from. Yet few people are aware that certain fats can actually help you lose weight. Ann Louise Gittleman in her book *Beyond Pritikin*, tells how she discovered that while her female patients were given evening primrose oil supplements for PMS problems, they were pleasingly surprised to find that they were losing weight as well. She did some investigation and found that the right kind of fat actually stimulates a process in the body that burns available tissue fat. Gamma linolenic acid (GLA), an essential fat, not only has been shown to activate the body to burn fat, but to improve cardiovascular conditions and a number of problematic hair, skin, and nail conditions as well. With small amounts of these helpful fats, appetite normalizes, body weight stabilizes, and calories burn more efficiently. When these factors occur, lasting weight loss can be a reality.[8]

A toxic colon can also lead to fatty deposits in the blood vessels, due to the fact that an unhealthy bowel will not eliminate cholesterol as well as a healthy one. And of course, diets high in animal fats and other fats high in saturates (including hydrogenated fats) tend to damage vessel walls and cause hardening of the arteries.[9]

The issue of cholesterol has been getting an incredible amount of press lately. Cholesterol deposits in the blood vessels decrease the diameter and flexibility of the vessel and, as mentioned before, force the heart to work harder to supply blood throughout the body. With the recent announcements that nutritional approaches can often control cholesterol levels in the blood, many people are hoping that restructuring their diets will help. More and more articles on the topic appear daily, not only in medical journals and health food publications, but in many national news magazines as well. *Time Magazine* even devoted a cover story to "good cholesterol" last year. The article, "Searching for Life's Elixir," explored HDLs (high density lipoproteins) and their relationship to prevention of coronary heart disease. Announcements by the Surgeon General of the United States have helped the public finally accept that nutrition is a key factor in maintaining a healthy circulatory system.

Earlier, while discussing fats, I explained how the "bad" LDLs deposit cholesterol on the walls of our blood vessels and the "good" HDLs actually remove cholesterol deposits from vessel walls. It has been shown that the ratio of total cholesterol to the HDLs in your blood is really the most determinant risk factor to heart disease.[10] Dr. Jeffery Bland, an expert in nutrition-oriented research projects regarding cholesterol and heart disease, states, "It appears we can prevent coronary heart disease by implementing a diet different than the standard American diet." He goes on to indicate that dietary change as simple as eating more natural foods, lower in fat and higher in dietary fiber and complex carbohydrates, can produce a noteworthy lowering of LDL cholesterol.[11]

In 1985, Scott Grundy, M.D., Ph.D., a leading cholesterol researcher, and a colleague, Fred H. Mattson, Ph.D., produced evidence that monounsaturated fats actually reduced cholesterol levels in the blood. This was exciting news since most scientists believed that only polyunsaturated fats reduced cholesterol.[12]

Recently, much research has been done on hormone-like substances in the body known as prostaglandins, which regulate metabolic processes throughout the body. They have been shown to regulate many activities on the cellular level, including immune response, inflammation, reproduction, blood-clotting, tumor growth, brain function, allergies, and blood pressure. These prostaglandins can only be produced from the two essential fatty acids, GLA, an Omega-6 fatty acid, and EPA, an Omega-3 fatty acid. In addition, the presence of hydrogenated or fried oils actually blocks the transformation of GLA and EPA into prostaglandins. Other factors known to block this process include aspirin, alcohol, radiation, high blood sugar, saturated fats, cholesterol, viral infection, and aging.[13] The discoveries of new benefits of prostaglandins have helped reverse the negative regard that the medical profession has had for fats.

Cardiovascular disease, America's number one cause of death, has been shown to be related to the intake of EPA and GLA. For example, fish oils containing EPA are known to reduce the stickiness of platelets in the blood that lead to blood clots, the cause of heart attacks and strokes. Fish oils also lower blood pressure and triglyceride (fat) levels in the blood. Researchers have found benefits from the use of prostaglandins in the treatment of pain in arthritics and in high blood sugar levels associated with diabetics. The prostaglandin PGA3 has been found to relax blood vessels, lowering blood pressure. Scientists are investigating the role of these substances in cancer prevention and treatment.[14] So many diseases are being linked to essential fat metabolism and the lack of prostaglandins every day that their value as supplements to our diets cannot be over-emphasized. Refer to Table 7.1 for detailed information on major fat types.

The popularity of oat bran as a supplement that helps reduce cholesterol problems in the circulatory system is due to the fact that it contains small amounts of GLA. By eating only one ounce of oat bran per day, you will probably lower your cholesterol level somewhere between 4 percent to 6 percent, according to Dr. William Castelli of the National Institute of Health. He also suggests that stabilized rice bran fiber may even be superior to oat bran in

Table 7.1 Basic Fat Types

Type of Fat	Sources	Comments
Saturates (saturated fats)	Pork, lamb, and beef fats; full-fat dairy products (i.e. butter, whole milk, ice cream, cream cheese), coconut, palm kernel, and palm oils; cocoa butter.	High in LDLs; contribute to plaque (include hydrogenated oils)
Monounsaturates (Omega-9)	Olive oil, avocado, peanut, high-oleic safflower oil, high-oleic sunflower oil, and canola oil.	High in HDLs; remove plaque
Polyunsaturates (Omega-3)	Mother's milk, fish oils, fresh flaxseed oil, soybeans, wheat germ, walnuts, pumpkin, leafy greens, chia seeds, fresh sea vegetables.	EPA, DHA (produce prostaglandins); protect cardio-vascular system, skin, bowels, immune system
Polyunsaturates (Omega-6)	Mother's milk, organ meats, lean meats, safflower, sunflower, corn, soy, cotton-seed,* sesame, legumes, raw seeds, raw nuts, leafy greens, spirulina, evening primrose oil, borage oil, and gooseberry oil.	GLA (produce prostaglandins); help burn body fat; reduce symptoms of PMS; strengthen cardiovascular system, hair, skin, nails, immune system

*Be careful—Pesticide restrictions on cotton are not as stringent as on other oil crops.

lowering cholesterol levels.[15] Rice bran has 21.7 grams of soluble fiber per 100 grams compared to 15.9 grams in oat bran.[16]

Other foods reported to strengthen the heart include buckwheat, asparagus, and hawthorne berries. You might want to substitute for foods high in saturated fats other items containing minimal saturates. Some examples include: tofu for meat, low-cholesterol mayonnaise for your current brand, and the varied soy products for dairy products. Your natural foods store personnel will help you to become familiar with all the tasty and innovative low-cholesterol products on the market today. Remember to check labels, as many products boasting low cholesterol may not be low in fat.

Sunlight, with all its negative press lately in its relation to skin cancer, can actually lower cholesterol levels in the blood. The more sunlight you get, the more cholesterol is brought to the skin surface and changed into Vitamin D. A two-hour sunbath can lower blood cholesterol levels by 13 percent.[17]

One important fact to be aware of is that cholesterol deposits mainly occur only in places where a break has developed on the inner lining (intima) of the arterial wall.[18] Because of the slightly abrasive action of the millions of gallons of blood that flow over this lining during a lifetime, it is important that proper nutrition be supplied to assure its resilience. Thus, the presence of cholesterol in the bloodstream is not as important as preventing a break in the intima through proper nutrition.[19]

The cells of a healthy intima undergo daily replacement. Certain nutrients are known to aid in this process, avoiding a breakdown problem and thus, avoiding accumulation of cholesterol deposits and other related complications. Dr. Irwin Stone, a world pioneer of Vitamin C research, maintains that a lack of Vitamin C and minerals, such as potassium and magnesium in the diet, can cause breaks to occur in the intima. These breaks become collecting points for cholesterol, lipids (fats), and calcium.[20]

In a healthy cell, the optimal ratio of potassium to sodium (salt) is 20 to 1. Due to the fact that in our culture sodium intake is usually 20 to 38 times above the needed amount, increasing our potassium intake and decreasing our sodium intake can greatly benefit cellular activity and thus the regeneration of the intimal lining of the blood vessels.[21] Kelp, soybeans, bananas, hot red peppers, garbanzo beans, and dried peas contain high concentrations of potassium.

In 1982, Dr. Trevor Beard of Australia conducted a scientifically controlled study involving ninety volunteers who were all taking medicine that had brought their blood pressure into a normal range. Half were randomly assigned to a group that followed a special high-potassium, low-sodium diet; the other half made up a group that didn't. Everything else in both groups was the same and the doctors and nurses did not know who was in which group. In the high-potassium group, four out of five patients were able to reduce their medication and one out of three was completely able to stop taking any drugs by the end of the twelve-week study! In the control group, less than one out of ten was able to stop taking their medicine. (The reason the control group showed any improvement is attributed to the extra blood pressure measurements and attention to health associated with participating with the study.[22])

Adequate magnesium, as I have mentioned, is also a necessary ingredient in maintaining healthy arterial lining. Some factors contributing to magnesium deficiencies include low hydrochloric acid in the stomach, a high-protein diet, a diet high in dairy products, and a diet high in refined foods. Vitamin C, as I mentioned, is also essential to a healthy intima. In the condition known as scurvy, which is caused by an extreme deficiency of Vitamin C, all such connective tissue breaks down.[23] Foods high in magnesium include kelp, wheat germ, wheat bran, almonds, cashews, and soybeans.

Exercise can be a significant factor in maintaining a healthy heart. Heavy exercise over many months will not only cause the heart muscle to become stronger, but will even cause more blood vessels to be built to the heart to increase its food supply. This allows the heart to pump more blood per beat and beat less often to perform its functions. Because the heart does not have to exert as much effort in its daily workload, this also can decrease the risk of heart attacks.[24] Of course, if you have a heart problem you should consult with your doctor to determine the exercise program that is best for your particular condition.

Research at the American College of Cardiology in Washington, D.C. showed that patients with existing plaque (cholesterol deposits in the arteries) were able not only to halt the progression of disease, but actually turn it back after starting a program of nutrition modification, exercise, and stress reduction.[25]

Supplements for a Healthy Heart

So now that we are more familiar with the importance of a healthy circulatory system and some of the influences, positive and negative, that contribute to its condition, I'd like to discuss which nutritional supplements are available to help us maintain a healthy cardiovascular system. Fortunately, there are several possibilities to choose from to sustain good circulatory nutrition.

Some Natural Products Used for Cardiovascular Nutrition:

☐ **Nature's Way North American Oat Fiber:** A supplement high in soluble dietary fiber that helps to reduce cholesterol problems in the circulatory system.

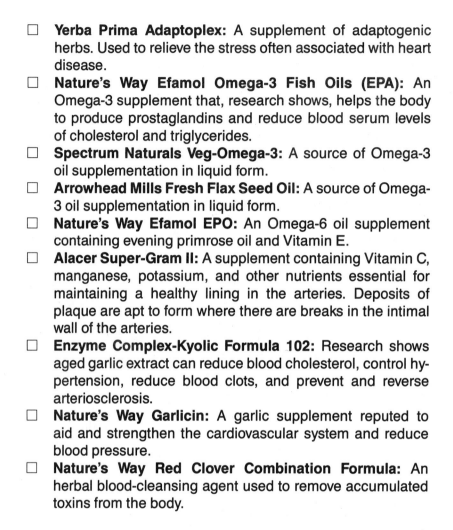

- ☐ **Yerba Prima Adaptoplex:** A supplement of adaptogenic herbs. Used to relieve the stress often associated with heart disease.
- ☐ **Nature's Way Efamol Omega-3 Fish Oils (EPA):** An Omega-3 supplement that, research shows, helps the body to produce prostaglandins and reduce blood serum levels of cholesterol and triglycerides.
- ☐ **Spectrum Naturals Veg-Omega-3:** A source of Omega-3 oil supplementation in liquid form.
- ☐ **Arrowhead Mills Fresh Flax Seed Oil:** A source of Omega-3 oil supplementation in liquid form.
- ☐ **Nature's Way Efamol EPO:** An Omega-6 oil supplement containing evening primrose oil and Vitamin E.
- ☐ **Alacer Super-Gram II:** A supplement containing Vitamin C, manganese, potassium, and other nutrients essential for maintaining a healthy lining in the arteries. Deposits of plaque are apt to form where there are breaks in the intimal wall of the arteries.
- ☐ **Enzyme Complex-Kyolic Formula 102:** Research shows aged garlic extract can reduce blood cholesterol, control hypertension, reduce blood clots, and prevent and reverse arteriosclerosis.
- ☐ **Nature's Way Garlicin:** A garlic supplement reputed to aid and strengthen the cardiovascular system and reduce blood pressure.
- ☐ **Nature's Way Red Clover Combination Formula:** An herbal blood-cleansing agent used to remove accumulated toxins from the body.

One prospect, which has been mentioned, is adding oat bran to your daily diet. This versatile item can be sprinkled over your cereal in the morning or combined with other food preparations. On the natural foods store shelves, numerous products can be found containing oat bran. Available are anything from cookies and chips to cereals, breads, and cakes of many different varieties. The only problem with these items is you don't always know just how much oat bran has been included in the products. Read the labels to see if oat bran is one of the first items listed. Ingredient labels must list items in descending order according to what percentage of the total product the particular ingredient contributes. In other words, the most abundant ingredient in the product is listed first, the second most abundant is listed second, and so on.

The best way to assure getting enough oat bran is to use straight oat bran, either as a grain to add to your food or as a supplement in capsule form. Many vitamin companies as well as herbal-supplement manufacturers carry a quality oat bran product in capsule form. Nature's Way North American Oat Fiber is one of these fine products, containing a combination of both soluble and insoluble fibers. It is the soluble oat bran fiber that has been shown to reduce cholesterol levels, and this combination contains four times the amount typically found in oat bran. Remember that oat bran is not a cure-all and even dietitians, enthusiastic about oat bran, admit it is only going to benefit you if eaten in combination with an adequate nutritional program.

Because of the relationship between stress and heart disease, Yerba Prima Adaptoplex may be a good supplement to consider if stress is a predominant factor in your life. This product was discussed in detail in Chapter 6.

There are some excellent supplements to assure your getting essential fatty acids in your diet. One such product is Nature's Way Efamol Omega-3 Fish Oils (EPA). This nutritional supplement offers a polyunsaturated Omega-3-series fish oil containing 18 percent eicosapentaenoic acid (EPA) and 12 percent docosahexaenoic acid (DHA). Together these substances help the body produce prostaglandins and reduce blood serum levels of cholesterol and triglycerides, which, in turn, can reduce the risk of coronary heart disease.[26]

Another good supplement for Omega-3 fatty acids is produced by a health-conscious vegetable oil company, Spectrum Marketing. Spectrum Naturals Veg-Omega-3 is cold-pressed, fresh flax oil. Flax oil is an excellent source of Omega-3 fatty acids as it is 57 percent Omega-3 by volume. Because this is a fresh product, it needs to be kept refrigerated to maintain its beneficial properties. Sold in an 8.5 ounce totally opaque container to protect it from light, it has certain advantages and disadvantages over a supplement such as Efamol Omega-3 Fish Oils (EPA).

The advantage of Veg-Omega-3 is its cost. It is considerably less expensive than the EPA supplements found in capsule form. Another advantage is that while many fish oils have been reported to contain trace amounts of pesticides and polychlorinated biphenyls (PCBs), the flax in this product is organically grown and therefore should be free of these contaminates. It is also more stable than the EPA of fish oils. At the time of this writing, Spectrum Marketing was beginning its own production of Veg-Omega-3, which was formerly produced by the Omegaflo Company. Arrowhead Mills Fresh Flax Seed Oil, a similar product using certified organic flax seeds in a totally opaque container, is currently being produced by Arrowhead Mills in cooperation with Omegaflo Nutrition, USA.

The main disadvantages of bottled oils over an encapsulated form of the supplement are the lack of convenience and the taste. Though it does not taste bad as far as oils go, most people are not fond of downing a tablespoon of oil and prefer the soft-gel Efamol capsules. It can, however, be mixed in salad dressings, sauces, spreads, blender creations, or some other creative recipes.

Evening primrose oil is a rich source of two fatty acids: linoleic acid (LA) and gamma linolenic acid (GLA) from the Omega-6 series. Besides supporting the health of the cardiovascular system, this is a popular product for sufferers of premenstrual syndrome, who claim it helps relieve their PMS symptoms. As mentioned before, some individuals find that using evening primrose oil helps to burn excess fat. If you are looking for an Omega-6 supplement, Nature's Way Efamol EPO made from evening primrose oil and Vitamin E (added as an antioxidant) is an excellent product of the highest quality. This highly regarded nutritional supplement is a result of worldwide research efforts of Efamol Ltd. of England. It has been proven as an effective source of GLA in more than 120 clinical and medical studies in 15 countries.[27]

In order to maintain a healthy intimal lining in the arteries and thus avoid the breaks where deposits of plaque are apt to form, there is an excellent supplement I would like to make you aware of. Alacer Super-Gram II, mentioned earlier in this text, contains an adequate supply of Vitamin C, manganese, potassium, and other nutrients essential for intimal health, all in forms that are easy for the body to utilize. This product is well worth adding to your daily regime if you desire a sound circulatory system, as it will also strengthen and benefit the immune functions.

In *Garlic and Health*, Dr. Benjamin Lau discusses numerous research studies involving garlic and pays special attention to Kyolic Aged Garlic Extract. This research indicates that detrimental circulatory conditions have been improved with the use of these supplements. Studies have shown that daily supplements of Kyolic can reduce blood cholesterol, though it may increase in the first few months due to stored cholesterol in the liver being released into the bloodstream.[28] There also exist further indications that garlic can aid in controlling hypertension, can reduce blood platelet aggregation and fibrin formation (which can lead to dangerous blood clots). It has also been shown to prevent and reverse arteriosclerosis in test animals and to improve the HDL/LDL ratio in the blood.[29]

Kyolic Aged Garlic Extract may be a good supplement to add to your diet regime if you are concerned with the health of your cardiovascular system. Because poor diet often precedes cardiovascular problems, the Kyolic formulation I would recommend for this condition is Enzyme Complex-Kyolic Formula 102. This formula contains natural enzymes that allow you to utilize the aged garlic extract more efficiently and effectively. By the way, this superb product contains no yeast, sodium, or dairy products for those concerned with these dietary restrictions. Nature's Way Garlicin, another garlic supplement that I have previously mentioned, can also help with hypertension and offers nutritional support for the cardiovascular system.

At this point, I'd like to mention one other type of herbal category, the blood cleanser. Sometimes called a blood purifier, this term refers to an herb or combination of herbs that help to cleanse or detoxify the blood and cells. Since many sicknesses and diseases are a result of an accumulation of toxins in the body, these botanical preparations can be important in maintaining health, especially when recovering from illness. Of course, if you are suffering from a serious illness, you should always consult your physician before adding a blood cleanser to any treatment you are already receiving.

One excellent blood-cleansing agent is the herbal combination, Nature's Way Red Clover Combination. Consisting of an assortment of eleven herbs, this formulation can be of great benefit in removing accumulated toxins from the body as a whole. With these toxins out of the system, the body can work more efficiently and effectively to restore and maintain a healthful condition.

Circulation, Varicose Veins, and Hemorrhoids

Poor circulation is a common condition that many of us have experienced. The usual indications of poor circulation are coldness in the hands and feet. Often, poor circulation can be an indication of a deficiency of Vitamins C, E, or rutin (a bioflavonoid found in buckwheat).[30] An iron deficiency in women can lead to a lowering of the body temperature as well.[31] If poor circulation is accompanied by a condition where, repeatedly, there is a tingling in the arms or legs, such as when one of your limbs "falls asleep," it can indicate an extreme deficiency in Vitamin B-6. Cayenne pepper is known to stimulate the flow of blood and improve circulation to the extremities. Often, by taking a supplement of one of these nutrients or adding some buckwheat to your daily diet, you can bring warmth to your hands and feet.

Some Natural Products Used for Circulation, Varicose Veins, and Hemorrhoids:

☐ **Yerba Prima Nutrimental:** An herbal supplement of ginkgo biloba extract that, research indicates, has the capability of improving blood supply to the extremities. (tablet)

☐ **Nature's Way Ginkgold:** An herbal supplement of ginkgo biloba extract that, research indicates, has the capability of improving blood supply to the extremities. (capsule)

☐ **Miracle Salve:** An herbal salve used for the relief of discomfort of varicose veins.

☐ **Hyland's Calendula Oil:** A homeopathic oil used to relieve the soreness around the anus associated with hemorrhoids.

☐ **Hyland's Calendula Off. 1X Ointment:** A homeopathic ointment used to relieve the soreness around the anus associated with hemorrhoids.

☐ **Hyland's Hemmorex:** A homeopathic salve used to shrink swelling of hemorrhoidal tissues and give temporary relief from pain and itching.

☐ **Energy Medicine Hemorrhoids/Pile:** A homeopathic combination used to provide relief of the discomfort that comes from a hemorrhoidal condition.

It also stands to reason that if your blood vessels are narrowed or clogged, the blood moving through the extremities will be moving slower, heating the feet and hands less efficiently. Ginkgo biloba, the herb found in Yerba Prima Nutrimental and Nature's Way Ginkgold, helps to dilate the blood vessels, which gives better delivery of blood to the tissues along with better drainage of wastes.[32] We looked at this remarkable herb when we addressed the topic of memory, where it was found to help bring nourishment to another extremity, the brain. Nutrimental and Ginkgold are also helpful for people suffering from reduced blood circulation in other parts of the body. Cold feet and hands, as well as heaviness and tingling in the arms and legs, can be nourished by allowing an adequate supply of oxygen and nutrients into these areas, a task that Ginkgo does quite well.[33] This support can result in a more comfortable and active lifestyle for many people.

The veins are thinner-walled and less muscular than the arteries. They rely to a great extent on the movements of adjacent muscles to move the blood through the veins on its journey back to the heart. The veins contain small valves along their length to prevent backflow of blood. When these valves break down, varicose veins result. Varicose veins are easier to prevent than to correct, but there are some measures that can be taken that may improve this condition.

Some research suggests that varicose veins are often linked to constipation. Varicose veins develop in response to a backup of blood. When we strain because of difficulty with constipation, the straining blocks off veins used for the return of blood from the legs.[34] Some of the measures already discussed for dealing with constipation may help prevent or improve problems with varicose veins.

Lack of exercise is also associated with the formation of varicose veins. Since, as explained above, the veins depend on the movement of muscles to move the blood through them, it only stands to reason if we are not moving the muscles in the legs, we stand the chance of developing a varicose condition. Simple walking turns the calf muscle into a "second heart," pumping blood upwards. Even some people who walk quite a bit don't receive the full benefit of this exercise because they wear high heels, which interfere with the natural contraction of the calf muscles.[35] Make sure you are getting enough exercise in low-heeled shoes (or even bare feet) to help prevent this condition.

Vitamin-E supplements used over a long period of time have shown some improvement for sufferers of varicose veins. Drs. Evan and Wilfrid Shute reported many cases of improvement in this condition when 400 to 800 I.U. doses were administered daily. Some research in France has shown improvement of varicose conditions with bioflavonoid supplements.[36]

One product that has benefited many sufferers of varicose veins is produced by a cottage industry in Colorado. The product is called Miracle Salve by Miracle Products Company. Made exclusively for the relief of discomfort from varicose veins, it is an herbal salve that is applied externally to the affected area. I have yet to find a product that is produced by one of the more sophisticated manufacturers that works as well. Numerous testimonies from the many satisfied customers who swear by this product are enough to warrant mentioning it here. Continued use three to four times daily is recommended.

Another problem associated with veins, sometimes brought on by constipation, is hemorrhoids. According to conservative estimates, half of American adults over the age of forty suffer from this uncomfortable condition.[37] While most veins contain valves to prevent the backflow of blood, the veins in this area of the abdomen do not contain check valves. Gravity itself imposes a load on these delicate veins. In addition, if we are straining with our stools, pressure builds up in the rectal area and the blood backs up.

One product that may help relieve the soreness around the anus associated with hemorrhoids is Hyland's Calendula Oil. This product is a homeopathic solution, which can help soothe and heal irritations such as these. It contains extract of calendula (marigold), which is one of my favorite healing agents. I have seen, on so many occasions, how quickly it can heal many different types of lesions with frequent applications. Some may prefer Hyland's Calendula Off. 1X Ointment because a salve is sometimes more convenient to use, but I feel the oil is a little stronger than the ointment and, thus, a bit more effective.

Another Hyland's product that is specifically for hemorrhoidal problems is a homeopathic salve known as Hyland's Hemmorex. Hemmorex helps shrink swelling of hemorrhoidal tissues caused by inflammation, and can give prompt temporary relief in many cases from pain and itching.[38] This ointment is comprised of four carefully selected remedies to combat the suffering associated with hemorrhoids.

There is still another homeopathic combination that is worth trying if you suffer from this problem: Energy Medicine Hemorrhoids/Pile formula. This product, by Dolisos, is taken orally and combines six effective homeopathic remedies to offer relief of the discomfort that comes from a hemorrhoidal condition.

8

The Reproductive System

The function of the reproductive system is simply to bring about the formation of new members of the species. In simpler life forms, this takes place with the division of a cell, but in the more evolved human species we have a two-sexed (male and female) system of reproduction (as if you hadn't noticed). When a single sperm from the male fertilizes a single egg cell of the female, the formation of human offspring occurs. In the female reproductive organs, this fertilized egg undergoes billions of individual cell divisions to produce the infant at birth. All the organs of the male and female reproductive system are designed to bring about fertilization, development, and nourishment of the new offspring.

The male reproductive system consists of two external organs, the penis and the scrotum. Within the scrotum are the two male gonads (testes), where the sperm and the male sex hormone testosterone are produced. The penis has the ability to become fixed and erect in times of sexual stimulation, which facilitates its penetration into the female vagina during intercourse. Within these organs are a series of tubes, ducts, and glands that allow the semen containing the sperm to pass into the vagina, allowing fertilization of the female egg.

The female system consists of the female gonads or ovaries (from the Latin *ovum* meaning egg). The ovaries produce and secrete the female sex hormones estrogen and progesterone and the reproductive cells or eggs. The ovaries are two oval organs about 1.5 inches in length and are located in the upper part of the pelvic cavity on each side of the uterus. The uterus is a thick-walled, pear-shaped organ where the fertilized egg can implant. It provides an environment for the development of the fetus. Each month, an egg from one of the two ovaries is released, via one of the two fallopian tubes, to the uterus. Sperm enter the uterus through the vagina during intercourse. The vagina is a tubular canal, four to six inches long, which functions both as an organ of copulation and a birth canal when a baby is ready to be born. The mammary glands are considered accessory reproductive glands, providing breast milk for the nourishment of the newborn.

The menstrual cycle (from *menses*, the Latin word for monthly) normally occurs in females around the age of thirteen and continues on a fairly regular basis, every twenty eight days, for approximately thirty five years. This cycle begins with the onset of menstrual flow, known as the menstrual phase, and lasts for about four days. When the ovum is not fertilized, estrogen and progesterone secretion decreases, resulting in the disintegration of the endometrial lining of the uterus. This disintegration includes some bleeding, which drains from the body through the vagina. From the fifth day to about the fourteenth day of the cycle, the proliferative phase occurs and is characterized by estrogen stimulation. At approximately the fourteenth day, the secretory phase begins and ovulation occurs. Ovulation is the releasing of an ovum (egg) from the ovary and is accompanied by the secretion of several hormones that help prepare the uterine wall for implantation of the ovum, should it become fertilized. This phase continues until the twenty-eighth day when the cycle repeats itself.

Many common problems associated with the reproductive system can be reduced or eliminated with proper nutrition or correcting emotional imbalances. Unfortunately, due to a lack of understanding, much suffering is endured, especially by women who feel there is no easy cure for their conditions.

Female Problems

Every month, millions of American women will experience the unfortunate condition known as PMS (premenstrual syndrome). Sometimes referred to as pre-MONSTER-al syndrome, this uncomfortable condition may result in psychological complaints such as irritability, restlessness, impatience, depression, lethargy, fatigue, insomnia, indecisiveness, dizziness, nervousness, anxiety, and mood swings. Physical symptoms may include edema (retaining of water), lower abdominal pain (including cramps), constipation, headaches, weight gain, sweet cravings, breast tenderness, and bloating. In all, researchers have claimed to have identified 150 symptoms of PMS. Just prior to the menstrual period, women may be more susceptible to illness, allergies, and accidents, while being less tolerant to pain and stress.[1]

Most studies suggest that 30 percent of the female population suffers from PMS, but some authorities report that as high as 80 percent of women are affected by one or more of these symptoms.[2] From 30 to 40 percent of women experience symptoms severe enough to interfere with normal activities and lifestyle, and about 10 percent have symptoms so severe that they are considered disabled or incapacitated for several days of each cycle.[3] Premenstrual syndrome begins about one week before menstruation and usually is present until just after the onset of the menstrual flow. PMS is not directly related to painful menstruation (cramps), as a woman may suffer either from one problem alone or both together.[4] It is most common in women between the ages of 30 and 49, who had mothers with PMS, and who have irregular menstrual cycles. PMS is most likely to begin or become more severe after major hormonal changes such as pregnancy, tubal ligation, or discontinuing birth control pills.[5]

The exact cause of PMS has not been determined. Some of the proposed causes include improper estrogen/progesterone ratio, excessive swings in hormone levels, prostaglandin imbalances, and an imbalance in the brain's neurotransmitter chemicals. Because of the wide range of symptoms involved and the individual nature of each case, it is probably related to a series of imbalances rather than a single problem.[6] Dr. Janet Zand says studies show that women who suffer from PMS consume at least 50 percent more refined carbohydrates, sugar, high-fat dairy products and sodium than do non-sufferers.[7] This would indicate to me that good nutrition is essential to correcting imbalances associated with this widespread problem.

Medicinal approaches to treating PMS exist, including the use of hormones as well as prescription drugs. But there are also nutritional approaches that may prevent or alleviate the condition. Because much of the discomfort is due to water retention and because salt is considered a key factor in the retention of fluids, reduction of the amount of salt in one's diet may be of some help. Regular exercise has been shown to help reduce premenstrual symptoms as well.

Vitamin B-6 is also recognized as a useful supplement for PMS symptoms. Also known as pyridoxine hydrochloride, it is generally regarded as a safe, natural diuretic. The recommended dose is 100 milligrams, 3 times a day, starting about 10 days before the cycle.[8] A study using doses of 200 to 800 milligrams daily showed a significant improvement of PMS symptoms in a majority of women.[9] It also led to a decrease in serum estradiol, and an increase in serum progesterone, which is considered a favorable hormonal shift.[10] It is advisable to supplement your diet with a strong B-Complex formula when taking large doses of B-6, just to keep your system in balance. It is not necessary to take as much of the B-Complex as the dosages of B-6, however. Some women find extra niacinamide, one of the B-complex vitamins, helps control some of the emotional oversensitivity that accompanies PMS.

Some researchers have also discovered that women suffering from PMS show a deficiency of magnesium in their system.[11] In studies combining B-6 with magnesium, improvement of PMS symptoms was reported, apparently because the B-6 helped the magnesium ions to enter the muscle cells of the uterus. Due to the antispasmotic effect of magnesium in muscle tissue, it is conceivable that uterine cramps might be reduced.[12] Because magnesium works in conjunction with calcium in the body, one might want to add a supplement of these minerals to their diet as well. A generally recommended daily dose of these minerals is 800 milligrams of calcium and 400 milligrams of magnesium.[13] Many doctors recommend a calcium/magnesium supplement with added zinc as the best mineral combination for PMS problems.

Some Natural Products Used for Female Problems:

☐ **Yerba Prima Dong Quai:** A supplement of an Oriental herb traditionally used for female problems. (tablet)

☐ **Nature's Herbs Don Quai:** A supplement of an Oriental herb traditionally used for female problems. (capsule)

☐ **Zand PMS Herbal:** An herbal combination formulated as a supplement to the female system and used by sufferers of premenstrual syndrome (PMS) symptoms.

☐ **Nature's Way Efamol EPO:** A supplement of evening primrose oil that has brought relief to many women suffering from PMS.

☐ **Zand Female Formula:** A nutritional formula for women to use during the menstrual period.

☐ **Yerba Prima Colon Care Formula:** Dietary fiber has been shown to have a relationship to a harmonious menstrual cycle.

☐ **Natra-Bio Bladder Irritation:** A homeopathic preparation used to provide relief for symptoms of occasional minor bladder irritation accompanied by frequent, scanty, or painful urination.

☐ **Nature's Way Primadophilus:** *Lactobacillus acidophilus* has been shown to improve some candida conditions.

☐ **Yerba Prima Fiberdophilus:** *Lactobacillus acidophilus* has been shown to improve some candida conditions.

☐ **Living Source Complete B-Complex Nutrient System:** An excellent B-Complex vitamin supplement made with low-potency Food Grown nutrients.

☐ **Nature's Way Caprinex:** Research shows that caprylic acid has the ability to effectively stop the growth of *Candida albicans.*

☐ **Nutrapathic D-Yeast:** A natural supplement that works to bring the level of candida proliferation back to a normal harmless population.

☐ **Nutrapathic Nutra-Mune:** A synergistic combination of vitamins, minerals, amino acids, glandulars, herbs, and digestive aids developed to assist Nutrapathic D-Yeast (see above) by providing nutritional support to the immune system.

☐ **Flora Balance:** A liquid consisting of *Bacillus laterosporus,* protein, vitamins, and minerals, which quickly destroys candida organisms in the intestinal tract, restoring normal intestinal flora destroyed by *Candida albicans.*

☐ **Nature's Way Change-O-Life Formula:** A balancing herbal supplement for use during times of hormonal stress such as menopause and puberty.

Dong quai is a native Chinese plant that has been used for many centuries as a supplement for many female conditions. Dong quai is good for feeding the body's endocrine glands and for providing strength to women's glandular functions.[14] It is considered a "blood builder" as it contains both iron and Vitamin E. I mentioned this botanical earlier for treatment of tension headache because of its ability to relax muscles, and many women find this property comes in handy when muscle spasms cause painful menstrual cramping. Yerba Prima Dong Quai is a high-quality, standardized supplement, in tablet form, made from this herb. Nature's Herbs Dong Quai is also an excellent capsulated supplement of this botanical. I have known women who have taken this herbal regime for several months and have been delighted to find their uncomfortable premenstrual and menstrual symptoms reduced significantly. They reported that taking one tablet daily, increasing this dose to two tablets one week before menstruation, and to three tablets during the menstrual period had given them their beneficial results.

A number of natural PMS formulas are available. But the one I would be most apt to recommend is Zand PMS Herbal. This wonderful formula was developed by Dr. Janet Zand using her knowledge of Chinese and Western medicines, and has shown favorable results for years in her clinic. Among other ingredients, this formula includes magnesium, Vitamin B-6, and dong quai. Another herb, bupleurum, is also included. Bupleurum contains *saikosaponins,* which are reported to reduce inflammation and ameliorate stress response.

Another product that was mentioned in an earlier chapter concerned with heart nutrition has brought relief to many women suffering from premenstrual syndrome. Nature's Way Efamol EPO is an excellent dietary supplement for this condition. Efamol EPO contains evening primrose oil and natural Vitamin E as an anti-oxidant. Evening primrose is a good source of Omega-6 fatty acids, the precursers of prostaglandins, which are so important to the proper functioning of every cell of the body.[15] Some women even find they lose weight while taking evening primrose, a wonderful fat-burning side effect of the oil of this plant. Backed by 120 medical and clinical studies in 15 countries, Efamol EPO is a product one can use with confidence.

Vitamin C, niacin, and rutin are all good supplements that can offer some relief for problems associated with cramping. It is suggested that these nutrients be taken daily, one week prior to menstruation.[16] Zand Herbal Formulas also produces a formula for use during the menstrual period. Zand Female Formula consists of extracts of the herbs dong quai and red raspberry leaf (long recognized in Western herbal medicine as the "female" herb). Both of these herbs are wonderful nutritional supplements for menstrual support.

One other item to mention: dietary fiber has been shown to have a relationship to a harmonious menstrual cycle by modifying estrogen metabolism, possibly in the intestines and in the liver. The greater the intake of fiber, the lower the blood levels of estradiol (the unfavorable estrogen).[17] Yerba Prima Colon Care Formula, which I have discussed in length when dealing with colon problems, is an excellent fiber source.

Another condition sometimes related to the reproductive system, which affects women more often than men, is the problem of bladder infections or irritations. The reason why females suffer from this ailment with greater frequency than males is a matter of physiological construction. The urethra is the tube through which urine leaves the bladder to be excreted from the body. Women's urethras are only 1–2 inches long while men's are 8–12 inches long. One reason women are more prone to bladder infections is that it is easier for bacteria to reach a woman's bladder. Some other factors that may contribute to bladder irritations include spicy foods, alcohol, birth control pills, caffeine, too much refined starch and sugar, food allergies, and foods high in oxalic acid (spinach, rhubarb, chocolate).[18]

Of course, severe bladder problems should be attended to by a qualified physician. There is, however, a homeopathic product that is worth consideration if bladder irritation is causing you discomfort. Natra-Bio Bladder Irritation is a combination of four natural homeopathic remedies designed to help with bladder problems. This product has been known to provide relief for symptoms of occasional minor bladder irritation accompanied by frequent, scanty, or painful urination.[19] If you are concerned with the side effects of antibiotics, and your bladder condition does not warrant a doctor's attention, you might want to give Natra-Bio Bladder Irritation a try.

Another bothersome problem that affects many women is the condition commonly called a yeast infection. Yeast infections are not actually caused by yeasts, but rather by a yeast-like fungus organism known as *Candida albicans*. The condition, sometimes simply called candida, is properly known as candidiasis. The organism that causes candidiasis is found on the skin of healthy people and rarely becomes a problem unless some predisposing factor is present. When it is eradicated by pharmaceutical medicines, it is likely to return unless the underlying environmental or metabolic factor is corrected.

One of the most frequent factors contributing to candidiasis is the use of antibiotics. When we employ a strong antibiotic to fight a bacterial infection, we tend to upset the microbial balance in some areas of the body. Beneficial intestinal flora can be eradicated by antibiotics, upsetting the balance in the colon. The sensitive environment in the vagina can also be altered so the undesirable *Candida albicans* can flourish. Often when this condition is arrested it reoccurs when antibiotics are again ingested. Diabetes, diagnosed or not, is another factor that may encourage vaginal infections. Other factors contributing to this problem include excessive sweating and moisture, and some speculate the wearing of pantyhose and nylon underpants creates a highly favorable condition for candidiasis to occur.[20] Over-indulgence in sugar is also thought to encourage a candida condition.

Leading immunologists estimate that 80 million Americans, both men and women, have some type of candida condition. Symptoms of *Candida albicans*, which may inhabit intestinal organs as well as other parts of the body, can mimic more than 140 different disorders. The simple organism when out of control can cause such symptoms as allergies, depression, hypoglycemia, menstrual irregularities, headaches, and fatigue—just to name a few.[21]

There are many women who have cured candidiasis with nutritional therapies though it is suggested that anyone suffering from this condition consult a doctor, as there is some danger (slight, but real) that these infections can worsen and become systemic. Jonathan V. Wright, M.D., of Kent, Washington, reported that he had success in curing candidiasis with a concentrated mixture of lactobacillus acidophilus and yogurt. The mixture is injected into the vagina following applications of anti-yeast medicine. Dr. Wright also found that in very early vaginal infections frequent applications of this mixture may correct the condition without the use of the medication.[22] There are also some reports of women curbing this condition by taking frequent doses of acidophilus culture in pill form. Nature's Way Primadophilus and Yerba Prima Fiberdophilus are two good acidophilus supplements mentioned in an earlier part of the book.

There are some cases of the correction of candidiasis with B-complex vitamins, as well.[23] If you are considering supplementing your diet with B vitamins, I would recommend the low-potency "food-bound" variety found in Living Source Complete B Complex Nutrient System. I spoke about the excellence of this Rainbow Light product in detail under the topic of stress.

There is also a great deal of clinical research validating that caprylic acid has the ability to effectively stop the growth of *Candida albicans*. Caprylic acid is a fatty acid found naturally in coconuts and other foods, and is produced in small amounts in the body. Sodium caprylate is the solid salt of the caprylic acid and is readily soluble in water and thus more readily available to the body. The *Federal Register* of May 25, 1982 states that "The (sodium) caprylates have *in vitro* antimicrobial activity against dermatophytes (skin-borne fungi), *Candida albicans*, and bacteria."[24] One product that takes sodium caprylate and surrounds it in a cellulose fiber coating to offer a sustained-release action throughout the intestinal tract is Nature's Way Caprinex. Caprinex is a dependable, safe, and effective product for fighting candida infestations throughout the body.

Nutrapathic D-Yeast is another product of which sufferers of candida imbalance should be aware. I know one woman who had candida problems off and on for years and had tried both natural and pharmaceutical products to control the condition.

Her praise of this product is what first inspired me to investigate it. She told me she had experienced relief quite quickly after taking D-Yeast and that it was the best remedy she had ever found.

Nutrapathic D-Yeast works to bring the level of candida proliferation back to a normal harmless population. This product, which contains some sodium caprylate as well as other natural components, helps to restore the balance of candida populations in the entire body including the colon and the bloodstream. The D-Yeast nutritional formula does not do an overkill on the yeast population, which may lead to an excess of toxins in the body. Instead it works with the body nutritionally to restore a balance.

We do have internal systems designed to control the levels of microorganisms in the body. When suffering from a candida condition, it is, therefore, important to strengthen one's immune system so the body's defenses can establish and maintain a balance of beneficial organisms. Nutrapathic Nutra-Mune was developed to assist D-Yeast with this function. Nutra-Mune is a synergistic combination of vitamins, minerals, amino acids, glandulars, herbs, and digestive aids that are bioavailable in the body. They work together to enhance the body's natural balance when stress factors occur. It provides powerful nutritional support to the internal defense systems weakened by pollutants and the presence of *Candida albicans*.

So if you do suffer from candidiasis, you might want to try the teamwork of "the Candida combo" from Nutrapathic as a possible solution to this problem, the D-Yeast to normalize the candida population and the Nutra-Mune to strengthen the body's natural systems that tend to keep us in a balanced healthy state. With a dose of only three tablets per day and no strict diet change, this combination has provided effective candida control for many sufferers.

Another product that has been used successfully in reducing *Candida albicans* cells is a colorless, tasteless, soy-based liquid known as Flora Balance. This supplement, consisting of *Bacillus laterosporus* culture, protein, niacin, Vitamin B-12, and a host of trace minerals, has the ability to quickly destroy candida organisms in the intestinal tract. This colonization results in the restoration of normal intestinal flora while destroying the *Candida albicans* organisms.

Bio-Genesis, the manufacturer, is producing the first product to be sold in the United States containing this spore-forming bacteria, indigenous to the human intestine. In Japan, this culture has been used as a supplement for some time. Laboratory and clinical tests conducted by the Candida Research and Information Foundation have shown that these spores effectively reduce the number of candida cells and that the most dramatic results appear to be in those cases with gastro-intestinal symptoms. In the lab tests, Flora Balance was shown to reduce candida plate counts in a 28-day period, by 99.8 percent![25]

Because this product is effective in killing yeast and fungus cells, 10 to 20 percent of people taking this product report having varying amounts of "die-off reactions." If you experience a mild discomfort from such a reaction, it can be reduced or eliminated by lowering the dosage and working up slowly to the recommended level of two tablespoons per day for adults and one tablespoon for children two to six years old.

One other excellent product for women to investigate is Nature's Way Change-O-Life Formula. This combination of seven synergistic herbs, formulated by the late Dr. John R. Christopher, can be a helpful balancing supplement during times of hormonal stress. A recent article in the *New York Times* revealed that researchers in Sweden have found that a hormone that menopausal women take in combination with estrogen may increase the risk of breast cancer. The study, conducted by Dr. Leif Bergvist of University Hospital in Uppsala, Sweden, involved 23,244 women who took hormones after menopause, one third of whom took the combination of progestin and estrogen. The rate of breast cancer in the group that took the combination of hormones was four times higher than among the group that took no drugs at all. The group that only took estrogen had a breast cancer rate twice that of the group that took no drugs. Millions of American women are taking this combination of drugs to relieve the symptoms of menopause and prevent heart disease and osteoporosis.[26] This is another case in point for opting for the safer natural alternative whenever possible. Supplying the proper nutrition to the female system on a daily basis may also make menopause a less-severe event when that time comes around. Change-O-Life Formula should be considered not only for menopausal problems, but also for teenagers (both male and female) dealing with the hormone-induced uncertainties of puberty.

Many female sexual problems, from menstrual cramps to frigidity, are a direct result of deep-seated psychological problems. These problems may be caused by guilt feelings induced by parents, clergy, or a sexual partner when dealing with the subject of sex. The attitudes of these influential people in an individual's life may have produced mental patterns that directly relate to physiological sexual problems. Traumatic events such as child molestation or rape can also produce sex-related problems. At any rate, in our society sex is often considered such a taboo that many individuals suffer from some sort of sexual inhibitions, which can be manifested as physical problems.

If the psychological problems are too severe, counseling from a qualified therapist may be the only solution. At the same time, there are some methods that may aid the normal sexual problems that are the result of mental conditioning. Mental affirmations, and the use of the many subliminal tapes available, may be of some benefit. Also, Louise Hay's book *Heal Your Body* offers several excellent affirmations for female problems such as frigidity, cramps, and PMS.

Male Problems

It would seem that males get off pretty easy in comparison to females, at least where having problems with their sexual organs are concerned. We are lucky not to have the inconvenience of a menstrual cycle interrupting our normal schedules every month. We also are not required to carry the responsibilities of pregnancy and birth, along with all the possible limitations and complications that are associated with these important roles. On the other hand, we can never know the mysteries of having a human grow and develop within us and the remarkable accomplishment of actually offering the foundation for a life to begin. Even though, on the physical level, we are not as involved as females in the propagation of life, we are still essential in this process; and, for this reason, it is just as important for men as women to maintain a healthy reproductive system.

Even though medical literature indicates that male sexual problems have always existed, they seem to have grown more common with the advent of modern technology. Poor nutrition and extreme levels of mental and emotional stress seem to contribute to this increase. Several nutrients are known to be vital for the health of the male reproductive organs including Vitamin E, zinc, and selenium. These nutrients are coincidentally among the most common to be deficient in the normal American diet.[27] Fortunately, there are some wonderful natural products available to supplement the diets of health-seeking males.

Some Natural Products Used for Male Problems:

- [ ] **Yerba Prima Chinese Ginseng:** A standardized herbal preparation used for nutritional support for the male glandular system.
- [ ] **Yerba Prima Siberian Ginseng:** A standardized herbal preparation used as an overall tonic and stress supplement for both men and women.
- [ ] **Zand Active Herbal:** A balanced herbal formula used as a tonic to build strength and endurance in active men and women.
- [ ] **Rainbow Light Male Toning System:** An herbal and vitamin formulation designed to provide nutrition for the male glandular system.
- [ ] **Zand Male Formula:** An herbal formulation designed to strengthen the male glandular system.
- [ ] **Nature's Way Bee Pollen:** Research shows that bee-pollen supplements can improve the condition of prostate sufferers.

An herb long renowned as the esteemed supplement for the male system is ginseng. Ginseng is the male equivalent of dong quai, which was discussed under female problems. It has been used traditionally for centuries in both Russia and China to strengthen the male glandular system and as a general promoter of health. The T'ang Dynasty of China prized ginseng enough to give it as royal gifts; and at times in history its value has been worth more than its weight in gold![28] It also has an application for both male and female athletes and other individ-

uals engaged in concentrated physical and mental work. But it
is not recommended for females to use ginseng during pregnancy, as it may cause a hormonal imbalance at this critical
time.[29] Though it is employed in Oriental medicine for its abilities to preserve health, invigorate the system, prolong life, and
treat numerous diseases, its main use is as a preventative
tonic.[30] Ginseng is also considered an adaptogen because of its
ability to normalize adverse conditions that may affect the body
(see Chapter 6).

There are three predominant varieties of ginseng on the market: Korean and Chinese (*Panax ginseng C.A. Meyer*), Tien-Chi
(*Panax Pseudo ginseng*), and American (*Panax quinquefolium*).
Panax means "cure it all" in Latin. There is another botanical
known as Siberian ginseng, which is not really a member of the
Panax genus, which makes up the true ginsengs. Though Siberian ginseng is classified in the *Eleutherococcus* genus, it earned
its name because it contains many of the properties of the *Panax*
herbs.

With over 1,400 scientific papers published on the subject of
Korean ginseng, there are no reports that indicate any adverse
effects of this stimulant herb except for mild insomnia in some
individuals.[31] For this reason it is advised that Korean ginseng
not be taken in the evening or before bed. Siberian ginseng also
has much scientific documentation supporting it, with over
1,000 studies showing its health benefits published in Russia
alone.[32] Siberian ginseng also does not seem to cause any adverse effects and it does not appear to cause the insomnia some
experience from the Korean variety.[33] Siberian ginseng is considered to be a tonic to the entire body as well, but is not as specifically oriented to the male system as the Panax varieties. Because of this, it is more desirable for use by females than the
Chinese and Korean varieties. Many take Siberian ginseng for
its adaptogenic properties that help to reduce the effects of
stress. Chinese ginseng is very similar to the Korean variety in
its makeup and its properties. Tien-Chi has similar properties,
but has not been researched as much and is not as widely used
as the other *Panax* varieties. American ginseng (also called Red
American ginseng), native to our southwestern states, has long
been used by the Hopi and Papago Indians and in our American herbal medicine. American ginseng contains complex

chemical substances known as anthraquinone derivatives, which can have a laxative effect when taken in sufficient quantities.[34] Nevertheless, the wild American ginseng plant is highly valued, but its prohibitive price (it is perhaps the most expensive herb available) makes it inaccessible to most people.

A wonderful ginseng supplement is Yerba Prima Chinese Ginseng. This product is a standardized herbal preparation available in the form of a comfortably sized tablet. Each tablet contains 50 milligrams of ginseng extract, 25 percent of which is the active ingredient found in ginseng, known as ginsenosides. Because ginseng roots are shown to display a wide range of quality, many people prefer to take a standardized product to ensure consistent dosages and results.

Yerba Prima also has a Siberian ginseng supplement in tablet form. Yerba Prima Siberian Ginseng was the first Siberian ginseng available that was standardized for strength and consistency.[35] Again, the wide variation in constituent levels found in this noteworthy herb make this a meaningful accomplishment; this feat was only recently mastered. Even though this product contains the exact amount of active ingredients needed for optimum benefits, it also contains the whole plant root so that the full spectrum of the plants' unidentified cofactors will also be present. Yerba Prima Siberian Ginseng provides an excellent overall tonic and stress supplement perfectly adaptable for both men and women.

One product that includes the toning capabilities of Siberian ginseng in combination with other outstanding herbs is Zand Active Herbal. This product was formulated during the 1984 Olympics by Dr. Janet Zand, and tested for effectiveness on world-class athletes, including runners, cyclists, basketball players, and hockey players by Dr. Whitfield Reaves.[36] This formula was tested extensively for over four years before being released to the general public. Medical research has shown that Siberian ginseng increases maximal work capacity, partially due to enhanced oxygen metabolism in the muscles.[37] American ginseng is also included for its toning and strengthening effects and the product contains no caffeine or other stimulants.

Active Herbal gives the extra edge in training, competition, and performance. But it is not just for athletes. Because it is such a well-balanced formula, it can be used on a daily basis by both men and women. It provides wonderful nutritional support for all types of active people. In the business world, it is ideal for those under stress and other work-related pressures. In play, it is a wonderful dietary addition for those who want to exercise to build strength and endurance.

Rainbow Light Nutritional Systems has formulated a fine supplement to provide nutrition for the male sexual system. Rainbow Light Male Toning System provides zinc, selenium, Vitamin E, as well as other essential nutrients from concentrated herbal preparations, essential for a healthy male glandular system. These nutrients are provided in what is known as their "Food-Grown" form, which research has shown is capable of allowing for greater absorption, retention, and utilization of nutrients within the body.[38] Because many who suffer with male problems also have a high blood pressure, the fact that Male Toning System contains no stimulants makes this product safer for these individuals. This product is not a cure for anything, but can offer a supplement for men whose problems stem from inadequate nutrition or undue stress. Rainbow Light's confidence in Male Toning System is reflected in the way it guarantees, with a full refund, that its customers must be completely satisfied with this product.

Another supplement for men desiring to strengthen their glandular systems, is the Zand Male Formula. The principal ingredients contained in this formula are Chinese ginseng, American ginseng, and an Oriental herb known as fo-ti. The properties of this herb are often compared to those of ginseng, though it has not been subjected to such rigorous experimental study. In the Orient it is said to improve physical and mental health, lower blood cholesterol levels, reduce high blood pressure and numerous other ailments and conditions.[39] The formula also contains other botanicals said to contain rejuvenating properties, such as gotu kola, damiana, and sarsaparilla. Combined with numerous other carefully selected herbs, Zand Male Formula is considered an "energy toner" when taken as a nutritional supplement on a daily basis.[40]

A problem every male should be aware of, especially after the age of 40, is that of an enlarged prostate gland. The prostate gland produces the fluid that acts as the vehicle allowing the sperm to flow into the female and fertilize the egg. Without the prostate gland to manufacture this fluid, the body can no longer transport sperm out of the penis, and because of this, the male is considered sterile. This gland is located next to the mouth of the male bladder and, if it becomes swollen, it pushes on the tube the expels the urine from the bladder (the urethra), interfering with its normal flow. Symptoms of an enlarged prostate gland include congestion and discomfort in the pubic area and/or a feeling of constant fullness of the bladder with frequent and urgent trips to urinate. As the problem progresses, the unconscious release of urine in small amounts can occur, forced out by a full bladder. As the urethra is interfered with to the extent that very little urine can escape, the urine floods back to the kidneys presenting the serious danger of poisoning the system.

When the prostate gland becomes this enlarged, normally it is removed surgically, leaving the man unable to father children, though it does not mean there is any lessening of his desire for sexual activity.[41] It is understandable, however, that most men are anxious to solve their prostate problems in a less-severe way.

There are some nutritional approaches that may help to maintain a healthy prostate gland. A German physician, Dr. W. Devrient of Berlin, did some research on pumpkin seeds and their relationship to prostate health. He noted that in Hungary, Bulgaria, and the Ukraine, where people eat pumpkin seeds in large quantities, there is almost no incidence of enlarged prostate or other prostate disorders. He postulated that a native plant hormone affects the hormone production in the body, which assists in maintaining a healthy prostate gland. Perhaps the protein content of pumpkin seeds, along with the unsaturated fatty acid content, may be responsible for the seed's reputation as a regulator of sex organs.[42]

There is evidence, as well, that zinc supplements may help prostate problems not involving infection or other serious problems.[43] The importance of this nutrient to sexual health in the male is reflected in the fact that the prostate contains zinc in concentrations ten times greater than in most other organs of the body. In a study at the Center for the Study of Prostatic Diseases at Cook County Hospital in Chicago, Dr. Irving M. Bush and colleagues found that 50 to 100 milligrams of zinc a day improved or eradicated symptoms in the majority of men complaining of chronic prostatitis (without infection) or benign prostatic enlargement.[44]

Some beneficial results were also reported by Gosta Jonsson, M.D., in the *Swedish Medical Journal*[45] using bee-pollen supplements in the treatment of prostate problems. With ten patients seen for at least one year, five became free of symptoms with no side effects being observed. In a similar study in Japan using the same bee pollen preparation, Yutaka Saito, M.D., found that treatment was "effective" in 29 out of 30 subjects.[46]

Nature's Way Bee Pollen is an excellent bee-pollen supplement that may be worth adding to your nutritional program. Coincidentally, bee pollen is the male seed in flowering plants. It also is considered to be one of the richest foods in nature, containing 19 of 20 known amino acids, 12 of the 13 commonly accepted vitamins including the entire B-vitamin series, and is 15 to 35 percent complete protein. It also is a rich source of minerals including calcium, phosphorus, magnesium, iron, copper, manganese, sodium, potassium, chlorine, and sulphur.[47]

As with female problems such as frigidity, impotence and other problems may arise in men from deep-seated psychological problems associated with the subject of sex. Affirmations such as the ones found in Louise Hay's book *Heal Your Body*, and the use of the many subliminal tapes on the market may help remedy these problems. Of course, if the condition is too severe, the assistance of a qualified therapist may be the only solution.

9

Muscles, Skin, and Bones

Three organs or systems contribute to the basic form of the human body. These include the skin (integumentary system), muscle (muscular system), and bones (skeletal system). Without any one of these, we would not be able to move around and experience the skills and talents that we develop over a lifetime. Without our skin, our skeletal system, or our complex system of muscles, our ability to experience life as we do would be extremely limited.

The integumentary system (skin) is an organ that covers the entire external surface of the body. It functions as a protective shield, keeping out bacteria and harmful substances. It also operates in the elimination of water and waste products and in temperature regulation (sweat). In addition, the skin functions as an organ of sensation. Tiny nerve receptors, sensitive to pain, touch, temperature, and pressure, found throughout the skin's surface, send signals to the brain, where the sensations are interpreted. Hair, nails, sebaceous glands (which secrete an oily substance to lubricate the skin's surface), and sweat glands are considered appendages of the skin.[1]

The musculature system is responsible for producing any and all movements of the body. External or action movements such as walking, waving a hand, or kicking a football are a result of coordinated contractions of our skeletal muscles. Internal or life-supportive movements such as the beating of the heart, the churning actions of the stomach, and the movement of the diaphragm in respiration are carried out by muscles known as involuntary muscles. Life would be a truly boring existence without the abilities provided by the body's muscles.

The skeletal system provides the rigid framework, which gives the shape and support to the body. It also serves the function of protection to the delicate and vital internal organs, including the lungs, heart, and brain. The skeletal system works in conjunction with the musculature system to allow the body to accomplish a wide range of movements. Two other functions of the skeletal system, which are not as obvious, include the manufacture of blood cells in the bone marrow and the storage of mineral salts, especially calcium.

Minor injuries to these three elemental systems of the body are common. The natural arena offers many fine products that can often help speed up the healing of such minor injuries.

Muscle Sprains, Spasms, and Bruises

There are several ways in which muscles and the tissues, tendons, and ligaments that connect muscles to bones can be injured. The most common occurs when there is a sudden twisting or stretching of a joint beyond the normal range of motion. This results in what is commonly known as a sprain, and is in reality a partial tearing of the ligaments around a joint. A similar injury known as a strain occurs when there is no tearing, but only a stretching of the ligaments.[2] Sprains can vary in severity from a slight injury to those causing serious damage around a joint. Severe sprains can be mistaken for dislocations or fractures as each of these injuries display similar symptoms. These symptoms include pain, swelling, and tenderness. Any serious suspected sprains should be immobilized, kept cool with an ice pack to prevent excessive swelling, and examined by a qualified physician.

Bruises are another muscle-associated problem, usually occurring from a muscle being struck with force. This may occur either from an external object or from a sudden jolt that brings a bone forcefully in contact with a muscle. The resulting "black and blue" appearance is due to the accumulation of blood in the tissues as a result of the rupturing of capillaries in the area.

Another problem occurring with muscles is what is termed a spasm. A spasm is a muscle that remains in a contracted state involuntarily.[3] This may occur after over-working a muscle in ways that it is not accustomed to. The muscle knots up and can sometimes be quite painful. When the main muscle in the front of the thigh (the quadriceps femoris muscle) is involved, it is commonly called a "charlie horse," a term that most of us have heard before.

Sometimes muscle spasms can be associated with other problems as well. Often when a vertebra in the spinal column slips slightly out of place, the adjacent muscle(s) may spasm, preventing the vertebra from easily returning to its normal position. Many of us are aware of how uncomfortable this condition can be.

When muscles are engaged in exercise, certain chemical reactions take place, leaving the waste products of this metabolism accumulated in the muscle tissue. After a strenuous workout, these waste materials build up faster than the body is capable of removing them from the muscles. The result is often experienced as muscle aches and pains at some point after working out. This is one reason the experts advise stretching exercises before and after strenuous exercise.

And finally another major cause of muscle pain is the tightness that occurs, especially in the area around the neck and shoulders, from our exposure to stressful conditions. This again illustrates the dynamic relationship existing between the mind and the body, discussed earlier in other areas of this book. The longer and greater the exposure to stress, the tighter and more painful the muscles can get.

Methods such as massage and particular products mentioned in the discussion on stress, can help us deal with stress-related tightness. Unfortunately, there are many individuals who have been so tight for so many years that having rock-like shoulders has become the norm. These individuals don't even realize how tight their muscles are. I'm sure if anyone has gathered the statistics as to how many Americans have never had a massage, even an informal one from their spouse or lover, the figures would be appalling. It is such a shame that such a wonderful vehicle is available to enhance our experience of life, and so many either don't recognize its potential or don't take the time to treat themselves to the luxury of feeling such relaxation. Besides massage and other methods that help deal with stress, there are also products that can help to ease and relax tight and spastic muscles that result from the intensities of life, as well as helping with other uncomfortable problems mentioned thus far in this chapter.

Some Natural Products Used for Muscle Problems:

☐ **Hyland's Arnica Lotion:** A homeopathic preparation used to aid the healing of bruises, strains, sprains, and tight or spasmodic muscles.

☐ **Yerba Prima Dong Quai:** An herb used for its antispasmodic properties to relax tight muscles. (tablet)

☐ **Nature's Herbs Don Quai:** An herb used for its antispasmodic properties to relax tight muscles. (capsule)

☐ **Camocare Pain Relieving Cream:** A salve used to provide deep penetration and relief for minor aches and pains of muscles and joints.

☐ **Breezy Balms Warm Up Rub:** A warming ointment used for relieving muscle aches and pains, or just to warm your muscles before vigorous exercise.

☐ **Energy Medicine Rheumatism and Muscle Fatigue:** A homeopathic formulation used to eliminate discomfort associated with overworked and tired muscles or to relieve rheumatoid-type symptoms.

☐ **Longevity Arthritis Pain:** A homeopathic formulation used to provide relief of arthritic-type symptoms.

☐ **Breh Athlete's Relief:** A bath salt with essential oils designed to relax and soothe tired muscles caused by overexertion and strain.

☐ **Breh Healthy Joints:** A bath salt with essential oils designed to reduce inflammation and pain caused by arthritis and rheumatism.

Whether you suffer from tight muscles, sprains, strains, bruises, or muscle spasms, there are a few fine products you should know about. These are the products I always reach for when I am faced with one of these discomforts. Hyland's Arnica Lotion is my first and favorite product dealing with injuries and stiffness of muscle and related tissue. I have seen, on so many occasions, such dramatic results with this product, that I highly recommend it for any of the conditions mentioned in the first sentence of this paragraph. Though it may not produce results 100 percent of the time, when it does I believe you will be as pleased as I have been with this healing aid. Often, when Arnica Lotion is quickly applied to a bruise, the pain and discoloring is reduced considerably. When muscles are tight or "knotted," application of Arnica Lotion often seems to "melt" the muscles, reducing the discomfort quickly and effectively. In the case of strains and sprains, it seems to effectively speed the healing process. One caution to note with this product is not to use it on an open wound as it can irritate an open injury.

Another product that works well with tight and cramping muscles is dong quai. Both Yerba Prima Dong Quai and Nature's Herbs Dong Quai are fine supplement forms of this herb. Dong quai, discussed in previous chapters, has antispasmodic properties.[4] This means it has the ability to relax muscles. This, in turn, can make it an effective tool in relieving the discomfort of muscles in spasm. I will often use dong quai internally while applying Arnica Lotion to the affected area externally.

Let me tell you two personal stories that I feel will demonstrate the effectiveness of these products. Once, many years back, I took a very lengthy mountain hike, an endurance feat to which I wasn't accustomed. The next morning I awoke to find both my calves knotted up to such a degree that I could barely walk. In fact, it was so painful to move around that I walked only to the medicine cabinet to get the Arnica Lotion. I applied it to my calves with a cotton ball and was totally amazed. Within moments, the muscles relaxed and I could walk around with almost no discomfort at all! This product does not always work this effectively or quickly, but often it does; and from that moment on, it has always been my first choice for similar problems.

One more story. One time I was taking a shower (I told you these were personal stories), and I twisted my body in such a way that I felt a vertebra in the center of my back slip out of place. For a day or two I tried to ignore it, as one side of my back started to turn into a large painful "knot." I tried stretching and hanging from a cross beam to try to pull things back in line, but nothing seemed to give any relief. Finally, I decided to take three Dong Quai tablets, morning and night, and at the same time apply Arnica Lotion to the affected area of my back.

Within a day and a half, with the muscles relaxed, the vertebra slipped back into place without an adjustment.

Camocare Pain Relieving Cream is another product worth mentioning. This product, made by one of the largest skin-care companies in Europe, is a unique formulation that provides deep penetration and relief for minor aches and pains of muscles and joints associated with arthritis, simple backaches, strains, bruises, and sprains.[5] In addition, because of the qualities of the chamomile herb, this soothing salve comforts tight and tender skin. This product can also be massaged into the skin before exercise to prepare and relax both skin and muscles. You may find that this precaution leaves you feeling less tense and tight after your workout.

If you are looking for a warming rub to use for relieving muscle aches or pains, or just to warm your muscles before vigorous exercise, Breezy Balms Warm Up Rub is a wonderful product. The deep heating action of Warm Up Rub provides a soothing effect on tight and painful muscles. This product does contain camphor, however, and therefore it is suggested that Warm Up Rub not be used with homeopathic preparations.

Rheumatism is a painful state of supporting body structures, namely bones, ligaments, tendons, joints, and muscles.[6] If we find ourselves suffering from rheumatoid-type symptoms, one natural product that may help bring some relief is Energy Medicine Rheumatism and Muscle Fatigue. This homeopathic combination, comprised of six individual remedies, has offered help to many sufferers of rheumatoid-type problems. It can also be helpful to eliminate discomfort associated with overworked and tired muscles.

Arthritis refers to many different diseases, all of which are characterized by inflammation in one or more of the joints. Inflammation, pain, and stiffness may also be present in adjacent parts of the body, such as the muscles near the joints. This condition can cause much discomfort and pain to the sufferer. The chronic pain that accompanies various arthritic conditions may be associated with the body's inability to produce endorphins,[7] which are naturally occurring painkillers, often produced when engaged in heavy exercise.

Because chamomile is known to relax muscle tension and ease joint tightness,[8] Camocare Pain Relieving Cream may offer some relief to those with an arthritic condition. Longevity Pure Products produces a homeopathic formulation, Longevity Arthritis Pain, which has provided relief to many sufferers of arthritic symptoms. This preparation consists of seven remedies for arthritis-related symptoms. The Longevity Company boasts of offering "user-friendly" homeopathy products. I really like their unique dispenser, which is compact, easy to use, and apportions the specified dose, without contamination, with a simple twist of the cap.

Two other products worth considering when suffering from sore or fatigued muscles or damaged joints are specially formulated bath salts from Breh. Breh Athlete's Relief is a combination of herbal extracts and oils designed to relax and soothe muscles tired by overexertion and strain. This formulation is also effective in helping heal minor injuries by warming, easing pain, and increasing circulation. Breh Healthy Joints is a similar preparation designed to reduce inflammation and pain caused by arthritis and rheumatism. This specialized bath salt formula helps cleanse and nourish the joints by enhancing circulation, digestion, and elimination. Both of these products utilize the principles of immersion therapy, herbology, and aromatherapy to induce their results. Both are combined with unrefined mineral-rich sea crystals to offer you a wonderful supplement to your hot bath. A good soaking in a warm bath is always helpful in such cases, and the addition of these products can only enhance the ability of a bath to ease the discomfort from muscle and joint problems.

Cuts and Burns

Minor cuts and scrapes are a common occurrence around the house, especially if there are children in the family. Cuts and wounds that bleed profusely should always be attended to by a qualified physician. Most minor cuts or wounds, however, can be safely dealt with at home. The first step should be to wash the wound thoroughly with soap and water. I always follow this procedure with an application of hydrogen peroxide to further sterilize the injury. When the injury is properly cleaned a healing agent can be applied.

Minor burns are another common skin injury. Burns are classified into three different categories. A first-degree burn is characterized by a reddening of the skin. Second-degree burns show a blistering condition has developed. And third-degree burns are characterized by deeper destruction. In the case of third-degree burns, the underlying growth cells that continually form new skin have been destroyed. Because of the lack of growth cells, third degree burns heal very slowly. The new skin can grow only from the edges of the burn area, where these cells can still function.

Third-degree burns and burns covering an extensive area of the body should be treated by a physician. Ten percent of the body affected by second- or third-degree burns is an extremely serious condition.[9] Even extensive sunburns can be considered serious. But minor burns (first- or second-degree) not covering large surface areas of the skin can be, and usually are, treated at home. Care should be taken when treating a burn, however, as damage can be increased due to the delicate nature of the burned skin.

Some Natural Products Used for Cuts and Burns:

- ☐ **Naturade Aloe Vera 80:** An Aloe vera gel containing comfrey that is used to soothe painful sunburn or treat other minor wounds.
- ☐ **Hyland's Calendula Off. Tincture:** A homeopathic preparation used to speed the healing of minor wounds that need to dry out.
- ☐ **Hyland's Calendula Oil:** A homeopathic preparation used to speed the healing of minor wounds that need to be softened or moistened.
- ☐ **Hyland's Calendula Off. 1X Ointment:** A homeopathic salve used to speed the healing of minor wounds that need to be softened or moistened.

Aloe vera is one herb that is renowned for its powerful healing qualities, especially when dealing with cuts, scrapes, and burns. One of the many fine aloe vera products available is Naturade Aloe Vera 80. This aloe gel contains 96 percent pure aloe along with a bit of comfrey added for additional benefits. Both herbs stimulate the growth of healthy skin and the aloe vera is also known to be a pain and scar inhibitor. This is a fine product to keep in mind when you want to soothe a painful sunburn or treat other minor wounds.

My all-time favorite healing product for both burns and other skin injuries is one form or another of calendula. Though many knowledgeable natural practitioners consistently recommend aloe vera products for burns, and I have used aloe gels myself for treating severe sunburns and other injuries with good results, I find calendula to work even better. *Calendula officinalis* is the Latin name for the common marigold. It possesses some of the most striking healing potential for skin injuries of any natural products I have studied or used. A powerful antibacterial agent that can prevent infection and promote healing, it inhibits the growth of bacteria, even on wounds that are badly infected, and is soothing as an external application[10] (though it may sting at first depending on the nature of the injury). It also has a tendency to stop bleeding when applied to a cut.

I always make it a habit to keep calendula around the house. This healing agent is considered to be a homeopathic remedy even though it is seldom used in the potentized form that characterizes most homeopathics. Oddly enough, you rarely see it mentioned as a healing agent in the herbal reference books.

I remember when I was first introduced to this product while taking a homeopathy course fifteen years ago. I was particularly impressed by the instructor's warnings that calendula not be put on a deep puncture wound without the use of another homeopathic remedy, hypericum. It seems that the healing action of the product can occur so quickly that the surface of the wound may heal up while infection may occur deep in the tissues where the calendula cannot reach. Hypericum is a homeopathic remedy commonly administered for infection.

Hyland's Calendula Off. Tincture is the same product I have personally used for over fifteen years and my confidence in it can not be expressed adequately. I remember being at work one morning when another employee received a small first-degree burn to his finger. I happened to have some Hyland's Calendula Off. Tincture with me and put some on his finger. He put a Band-Aid on it and went back to work. At the end of the day, as I was ready to leave, I asked him if he would like me to put some more on it. He took off the Band-Aid and, to his astonishment, the burned area was almost completely healed! On many occasions dealing with cuts, scrapes, and burns, I have seen other impressive results with this product.

Two other forms of this effective healing agent are also available. Hyland's Calendula Oil and Hyland's Calendula Off. 1X Ointment are similar products with their own merits. The usual rule as to when you might choose the oil application over the tincture, has to do with whether you might like to dry or soften a wound. Usually, a cut needs to dry out in order to heal properly while chaffed, windburned skin may require some moistening. Hyland's Calendula Oil is an excellent agent when moistening is the purpose trying to be achieved.

The advantage of Hyland's Calendula Off. 1X Ointment is that it is in a salve rather than liquid form, which can be convenient when transporting the product in a purse or suitcase. It is also in a plastic tube, instead of a bottle, which makes it safer for transport. In addition, it can be easier to apply and less messy than a liquid concentration. I don't believe it is quite as potent in its action, however, as the tincture and oil forms. Whichever form or forms you may choose to work with, I'm sure you will find it capable of relieving many problems associated with minor skin injures.

Skin Irritations, Bites, and Stings

Many different factors can cause irritation to the skin. Wind burn, minor scratches, rashes, eczema, chapped lips, chaffed or raw skin, diaper rash, skin reactions to household chemicals, and splits in the skin around the nails are just a few problems in this category. When we need to soothe irritated skin, there are many products on the shelves to choose from. Some may bring soothing relief, but at what cost? As we have learned, the skin can absorb most substances that are applied to it and if the product we are using has questionable ingredients, we may end up with harmful chemicals in our system.

Some Natural Products Used for Skin Irritations, Bites, and Stings:

☐ **Autumn Harp Comfrey Salve:** An herbal salve containing olive oil and wheat germ oil (rich in Vitamins A, D, and E) and used to relieve the discomfort and speed the healing of skin irritations, insect bites and stings.

- ☐ **Kangaroo Brand Australian Tea Tree Oil Lip Balm:** A moisturizing natural lip balm containing the healing properties of tea tree oil.
- ☐ **Desert Essence Jojoba-Aloe Vera Lip Balm:** A moisturizing natural lip balm containing the healing properties of Jojoba and Aloe Vera.
- ☐ **Hyland's Anacarium 3X:** A homeopathic remedy used internally for the prevention and relief of poisonous plant symptoms.
- ☐ **Breezy Balms Oak Away:** An herbal spray used to provide cooling relief from itching, swelling, and spreading of plant-induced skin irritations as well as insect bites and stings.
- ☐ **Boericke & Tafel Sssstingstop Soothing Gel:** A homeopathic gel used for relief from the pain, itch, and swelling caused by insect stings and bites.
- ☐ **Natra-Bio Insect Bites:** A homeopathic formulation used for temporary relief of the pain, itching, and swelling associated with insect bites.

One product that has safe, natural ingredients that I have seen some surprisingly positive results with is Autumn Harp Comfrey Salve. Recently, a truck driver came into my office after falling off the back of his truck a few days before. He had scraped a large area of his leg in the fall and it was beginning to become infected. I gave him a bottle of this product to try and he was so impressed by the results he received, he came back a few days later and ordered several jars.

This extremely effective medicinal ointment is made with the freshest organic herbs and the finest unrefined oils. The herbs are prepared on the same day they are harvested to assure maximum potency and freshness. They add unrefined, unbleached beeswax for consistency and gum benzoin as a natural preservative. Comfrey is an herb containing a substance known as "allantoin," which is a cell proliferant (promotes rapid regeneration of cells). Its astringent quality helps to draw infection from the body.[11]

Plantain, another herbal ingredient in Comfrey Salve, also has antiseptic and astringent properties, as well as styptic action, which helps to check bleeding.[12] Goldenseal, another component, is a non-irritating antiseptic that heals and soothes the injured surfaces of the body. The addition of olive oil and wheat germ oil as softeners and conditioners (rich in Vitamins A, D, and E) for dry and damaged skin help to round out this terrific formulation. Autumn Harp Comfrey Salve is a wonderful addition to your medicine cabinet. This product also fares well in the treatment of chapped lips.

Speaking of chapped lips, I would recommend Kangaroo Brand Australian Tea Tree Oil Lip Balm distributed by Desert Essence if you are looking for a good stick lip balm. The Australian tea tree has long been regarded for its medicinal properties by the Aboriginal people. The now-famous botanist Joseph Banks named it for the delicious tea that could be made from its leaves. In 1924, Drs. Penfold and Morrison of the Sydney Technological Museum investigated the unique properties of the tea tree species, *Melaleuca alternifolia*. Since that time considerable scientific work has been done on tea tree oil, leading to its widespread use in first aid, and dental and surgical practice in Australia.[13] The tea tree oil in this lip balm gives it an unusual flavor, but, at the same time, adds a powerful healing agent to the product. Australian Tea Tree Oil Lip Balm contains other healing ingredients including aloe vera extract, jojoba oil, and Vitamin E.

For those of you who don't like the strong flavor of tree tea oil, Desert Essence produces another, milder-tasting product. Desert Essence Jojoba-Aloe Vera Lip Balm combines pure jojoba oil and aloe vera to prevent and protect against chapping. Some lip balms leave what I feel is an uncomfortable thick, waxy layer on your lips. I prefer these two lip balms not only for their healing properties, but also because they seem to be less waxy than most of the competitive brands.

Another potential cause of skin irritations is contact with poisonous plants. The most common offenders are poison ivy, poison oak, and poison sumac. Nettles is another plant that can cause an uncomfortable reaction when it comes in contact with the skin. There are hundreds of other plants that can cause occasional cases of poisoning to sensitive individuals, but the four mentioned above are the ones an average person should know and avoid. The irritating substance in the poison ivy group is an oleoresin called urushiol and is contained in most parts of the plant. Symptoms occur a few hours to several days after exposure to the plant, and appear as reddening and blistering of the skin, usually with intense itching.

I was at one time very sensitive to poison oak. From my youth, I remember an embarrassing and uncomfortable incident after venturing off into the woods with a young lady friend. Ah yes, sweet and sour memories, including the itchy days that followed that frolic! Take it from me, there are certain places that you do not want coming in contact with these powerful plant substances!

Later, I discovered that there was a product available that was made of poison oak extract. One was to drink two small doses approximately two weeks before exposure as a preventative measure. As I traveled to an area of high concentration of poison oak several times a year, I would take this product a few weeks before I left on my travels and found I was almost immune to the effects of this plant. The few times I did contract poison oak it was very minor compared to symptoms I had gotten before I had access to this product. When I could not longer find the product, I contacted the manufacturer. Imagine my dismay when I learned the FDA had removed it from the shelves. Their reasoning, I was told, was that there was no clinical proof that it worked!

Now I take my chances with a homeopathic product, which I take before exposure. Hyland's Anacarium 3X is not as effective as the other product, but seems to be capable of building resistance, as well. Taking about five pellets per day starting approximately five days before exposure may also help build your resistance to the plant's poison. It also can sometimes be helpful in relieving some of the symptoms of poisonous plants.

In the event you do contract poison ivy, poison oak, or poison sumac, there are procedures and products that may improve the situation. First, if you suspect you have been exposed to one of these plants, take several showers with a good lather of soap each time, as soon as possible. Give your clothing a good strong laundering as well. The oils from the plant can be rubbed off on the clothing and then onto your skin and cause an irritation as severe as direct exposure. If it is too late and you already have been infected with a case of plant poisoning, it is a good idea to wash your clothes and bed sheets every day anyway, as the problem can spread to other parts of the body.

A helpful product for relieving the annoying itch is Breezy Balms Oak Away. This product contains nine helpful herbs in a base of sea water and alcohol. One of the herbs in this formula is jewelweed, a classic herbal remedy for poison-plant symptoms. Oak Away is a soothing spray (it comes in a fine mist bottle) that often provides cooling relief from the itching, swelling, and spreading of plant-induced skin irritations. My experience with this product has confirmed this. I developed a poison ivy-induced rash while hiking in the Rocky Mountains of Colorado. I sprayed Oak Away on the area several times each day and found almost no itching, no spreading, and a clearing up of the problem in a shorter time than I would have expected. Reports by satisfied users suggest that Autumn Harp Comfrey Salve can also offer some relief for symptoms produced by the poison ivy plant group.

Insects, as well as plants, can affect the condition as well as the comfort of our skin. Mosquitos and other biting insects can leave a small bump and a large itching sensation. The best product I have found for relief of the itching of insect bites is the previously mentioned Breezy Balms Oak Away. I was first introduced to this product when a sample was sent to me at the natural foods company for which I do purchasing. I was meeting with a broker who was scratching her legs while we talked. She complained of mosquito bites and I handed her the sample to try. She sprayed it on her legs right through her pantyhose and after a moment commented that she couldn't believe it, but all itching had stopped. Since that time I have used it repeatedly and have experienced similar satisfaction (without the pantyhose!). Autumn Harp Comfrey Salve may also help with irritations caused by insects as the alkaline makeup of one of its ingredients, the herb plantain, counteracts the acidity of insect bites and stings.

The sting of a bee can be a painful experience and there are some people who are so sensitive to the bee's venom that a sting can be life threatening. A little understanding of bees and wasps can help reduce the problems associated with stings.

Bees generally are not interested in stinging someone unless the bee is confronted directly in front of the hive or they get stepped on, squeezed, or caught in clothing or hair. When you get stung, the stinger shaft, a poison sac, and a tiny contracting muscle are left in your skin. As the muscle continues to contract, more and more venom is forced out of the sac and down the shaft into your body. If you can immediately remove the stinger, very little bee venom will enter your tissue. The trick is in knowing how to remove the stinger. The normal reaction is to grab the stinger and pull it out. The problem with this procedure is that you tend to squeeze the sac, injecting a lot of venom into yourself. The best way to remove a bee stinger is to scrape it out by scraping from the side along the skin's surface. The scraping can be done either with a fingernail or some other object such as the side of a pocket knife. The important thing is to accomplish this as quickly as possible. I have done this on several occasions when I used to keep bees, and because very little venom had entered my body, after an hour or so had passed, I often could not tell where I had been stung.

Another thing to know about stinging insects is that often when they sting you, they leave a scent that alerts other insects of their species to sting that area as well. Because of this, when you get stung, it is good to remove yourself from the vicinity as quickly as possible, just in case there is a hive nearby. This becomes more serious with wasps because they do not lose their stingers as bees do. Because of this, one wasp is capable of stinging an individual many times over.

An excellent application for relieving the pain, itch, and swelling caused by insect stings and bites is Boericke & Tafel Sssstingstop Soothing Gel. This pleasant gel not only provides temporary relief for the bites and stings of bees, wasps, fleas, horse flies, etc., but also for discomfort from nettle rash, hives, jellyfish stings, fever blisters, and cold sores.[14] Sssstingstop contains three homeopathic remedies to offer a cooling and soothing effect to hot, irritated skin. Furthermore, this preparation can be used as an insect repellent because it contains extracts of the aromatic herbs citronella and eucalyptus.

Another homeopathic worth mentioning is Natra-Bio Insect Bites. This natural formula consisting of four separate remedies for bite symptoms is taken internally instead of being applied directly to the bite area as with Sssstingstop. A few drops of Natra-Bio Insect Bites can offer temporary relief of pain, itching, and swelling associated with minor skin irritations, inflammation, and rashes due to insect bites.[15]

Bone Injuries

A fracture is a broken bone. Several degrees of fractures can occur. A fracture can be just a slight chip or crack in a bone. It can also be more serious, as in a complete bone break, a crushed bone, or even a compound fracture (when the broken bone protrudes through the skin). Even the slightest fracture can be painful due to the presence of many nerve receptors in bone tissue. When a fracture is suspected, the best thing to do is immobilize the area and have a doctor look at it. Quite often, a doctor will need to take an X-ray in order to determine the seriousness of this type of injury.

A Natural Product Used for Bone Injuries:

☐ **Hyland's Symphytum 12X:** A homeopathic remedy used to speed the mending of injured bones.

The only thing you can really do for a fracture is keep the affected body part still so it can heal correctly. A good product to use when you are recovering from a broken bone is Hyland's Symphytum 12X. This homeopathic preparation of the comfrey herb has been shown to speed the recovery of fractured bones. The herbal form of comfrey has earned the nickname "bone knit," due to its ability to speed the healing process of fractures. However, if you were to take a megadose of comfrey (which would be very hard to do), it would tend to make your bones brittle. For this reason, the minute potentized form of comfrey found in the homeopathic preparation tends to speed up the healing process.

10

Natural Care for Children

The best way to assure your child's health is to be healthy yourself. The diet and health of a pregnant woman, and even a woman in the months before conception, can have a great influence on the health and well-being of the child. The future well-being of your child can depend on the dietary choices you make throughout your pregnancy. According to noted pediatrician and author Robert S. Mendelsohn, M.D., most doctors know very little about proper nutrition because virtually nothing is done in medical schools to teach students that nutrition may often be the most important element in diagnosis and treatment.[1] Often obstetricians encourage the mother to stick to strict weight restrictions, which can persuade mothers to eat near-starvation diets the last two months of pregnancy, the period when the child needs maximum nourishment. Chances that an underweight baby will die during the first month of life are thirty times greater than those of a baby born at normal weight.[2] Fortunately, the issue of nutrition and the dangers involved with some forms of treatment are becoming more recognized by the medical profession as a whole, and many reforms have emerged within the last decade. But unless you are lucky enough to have a progressive, well-educated, nutrition-oriented doctor, it is the responsibility of expectant parents to educate themselves and use common sense when choosing the foods that will nourish their developing offspring.

After your baby is born, there is another important decision to make, whether to breastfeed your baby or not. Breastfeeding lays the foundation for healthy physical and emotional growth for development in infancy and for the rest of your child's life.

Mother's milk is nature's best nutritional formulation available. It not only provides all the essential nutrients the infant needs for the first six months of its life, but provides the natural immunity to many allergies and infections that is denied to bottle-fed babies. There are unique substances contained in mother's milk that inhibit the growth of bacteria and viruses, offering critical protection during the most hazardous months of your child's life.[3] In addition, the emotional development of both child and mother is enhanced by the bonding process experienced during breastfeeding.

One concern with infant formulas is the ratio and amounts of Omega-3 and Omega-6 fatty acids in their makeup. Dr. Neuringer, an authority on infant milk, recently expressed his concern at a "Dietary Omega-3 and -6 Fatty Acids" Symposium. He warned his colleagues about the low Omega-3/high Omega-6 content in infant formulas that can cause a serious imbalance among the resultant prostaglandins. These imbalances could impair the immune system and could dispose the infant to cancer and heart trouble later in life.[4] The concern is evident enough to motivate the Canadian equivalent to our FDA, known as the Health Protection Branch of the Canadian government, to consider requiring all infant formulas to contain adequate amounts of the Omega-3 fatty acid. Non-nursing babies can be fed a small amount of flax seed oil to provide the necessary amounts of these essential fatty acids.[5]

After the breastfeeding period is over, to provide proper nutrition for your child, follow the guidelines found in Chapter 3. A basic rule: the more a food product is processed, the less nutritious it becomes. Most foods are nutritious in their raw natural state, and as we tamper with them we tend to diminish their dietary value. You may want to consider feeding your baby some of the selection of organic baby foods now available at the natural foods stores. Raising your children on a healthy diet will build good eating habits for their adult lives. Try not to encourage their eating excess sugar. This may start with the habit of putting sugar on breakfast cereal or buying cereals heavily laden with sugar. Today, there are numerous tasty and attractive breakfast cereals with quality ingredients available in the natural foods stores across the nation.

Parents also need to learn when to call a doctor and when to treat the child at home. According to Dr. Mendelsohn, at least 95 percent of the ailments that children suffer will heal themselves and do not require medical attention.[6] He also claims that at least 90 percent of the drugs prescribed by pediatricians are unnecessary and a costly risk to the child who ingests them.[7] This is largely due to the fact that the doctors spend a great deal of their time treating parental distress when worried parents bring their ailing children in.[8] Dr. Mendelsohn's book, *How to Raise a Healthy Child . . . In Spite of Your Doctor*, is well worth every parent's time to read! His insight into the world of medicine and its effect on children is enlightening; his advice on when to call a doctor (and when to listen to them) is invaluable. His book will help you determine when medical attention is necessary and when an illness will most likely cure itself.

Natural Products for Children

Many of the products mentioned throughout this book are as safe for children as they are for adults, but labels should be read carefully to ascertain proper dosage levels. There are also some products that are designed especially for the needs of children. At this time, I would like to mention a few worthwhile quality children's products.

Some Natural Products Used for Children's Ailments:

- ☐ **Hyland's Colic Tablets:** A homeopathic combination that helps soothe and quiet babies with mild tummy aches.
- ☐ **Hyland's Teething Tablets:** A homeopathic combination that is used to help relieve the pain associated with the growing in of new teeth.
- ☐ **Kyolic Aged Garlic Extract:** An herbal liquid that is used as ear drops to relieve the pain of earaches.
- ☐ **Hyland's Bed Wetting Tablets:** A homeopathic combination that is used to improve this unpleasant problem when nothing serious is causing it.
- ☐ **Hyland's Calms:** A homeopathic combination that is used for relief of occasional sleeplessness and simple nervous tension.

- ☐ **Hyland's Cough Syrup with Honey:** A homeopathic combination that is used for relief of occasional sleeplessness and simple nervous tension.
- ☐ **Nature's Way Primadophilus for Children:** A culture used to supplement the beneficial intestinal bacteria in infants and children to age five.
- ☐ **Nature's Way Primadophilus Junior:** A culture used to supplement the beneficial intestinal bacteria in children between the ages of six to twelve.
- ☐ **Autumn Harp Comfrey Salve:** A soothing ointment used to relieve the discomfort that accompanies diaper rash and chaffing.
- ☐ **Bach Rescue Remedy:** A flower remedy used to instill confidence and calmness in a scared or injured child.

Colic is one problem commonly associated with infants. It is typically identified when a previously content baby suddenly draws up its legs and has a fit of screaming. This condition is usually attributed to mild indigestion and gas pains. Hyland's Colic Tablets have helped soothe and quiet babies with mild tummy aches for several generations.[9] If conditions persist or intensify, you should consult a physician, but these tiny homeopathic tablets, which melt instantly on the tongue, quite often relieve the problem.

Another discomfort babies, and their parents as well, are commonly confronted with is the pain associated with the growing in of new teeth. Because this process goes on for quite some time, it can be trying for both mother and baby. Hyland's Teething Tablets often help bring some relief to this difficult period. This homeopathic combination of natural remedies often relieves the restlessness, the whining, and the irritability caused by the teething experience.[10] This remedy is also often used to bring relief for earache problems in children.

Speaking of earaches, which seem to be a common occurrence with children, I think one product that may bring relief is Kyolic Aged Garlic Extract. The liquid form of this supplement (discussed in Chapter 5) has given many children relief, and some parents even report that it has lowered the frequency of occurrence of this disturbing ailment. A few drops placed in the affected ear and sealed with a small piece of cotton, twice a day, may help your child with this problem.

Bed wetting is a problem sometimes associated with an allergic reaction. It is interesting to note that bottlefed children are at least 20 times more susceptible to allergies than are breast-fed babies.[11] Whatever the cause, bed wetting is not only an uncomfortable and unpleasant occurrence, it sometimes can set up tensions between the parents and the child. If it isn't the child's fault, he/she still knows it's a problem for his parents. It is good to check with your physician to determine that nothing serious is causing this problem, and if not, Hyland's Bed Wetting Tablets are worth a try. For many years, parents and children alike have found this homeopathic preparation has helped with this unpleasant problem.

Hyland's also produces a homeopathic formula specifically for relief of occasional sleeplessness and simple nervous tension. This product is Hyland's Calms and is considered safe enough for use with children.[12] Calms is well worth being aware of when dealing with nervous or hyperactive children, or with normal children who have occasional problems with falling asleep.

One more product from Hyland's to be aware of is Hyland's Cough Syrup with Honey. This cough remedy is formulated especially for children, containing safe, natural ingredients in a pleasant-tasting honey syrup. It can be quite effective for minor coughs associated with a common head cold.

Children need to maintain healthy intestinal flora just as adults do. Sometimes this intestinal population needs to be supplemented to assure a proper balance of the beneficial bacteria. This is especially true if the child has been exposed to antibiotics, which tend to destroy the beneficial intestinal bacteria so vital to maintaining a healthy body. Because children need their own special formula and potency, two intestinal supplements are available for your child, depending on their age. Nature's Way Primadophilus for Children is a preparation specially formulated for children from birth to age five. It comes in powder form so it can be mixed in food or drink for children too young to swallow capsules. Nature's Way Primadophilus Junior is formulated for children between the ages of six to twelve. It comes in a smaller, easy to swallow "enteric-coated" capsules, designed to pass all the way to the intestines before being digested. Both offer the same quality as adult-strength Primadophilus, but in a form, formula, and potency suitable for each age group. These products are both hypoallergenic and contain no milk, soy, corn, wheat, yeast, or chemical preservatives.

I also feel it appropriate to again mention a product I described in detail when speaking about skin irritations. This product should be considered as a soothing ointment when dealing with diaper rash and chaffing. Autumn Harp Comfrey Salve is a powerful, yet gentle, natural medication. It has provided relief for many a baby who has suffered soreness resulting from damp diapers.

When a child is scared, in pain, or in a state of hysteria due to an injury, even a minor scrape, Bach Rescue Remedy can often help to instill confidence and calmness. If you try this flower remedy sometime, don't be surprised to see the child's mental state quickly return to normal.

11

Your Home
Medicine Cabinet

Now you have a virtual arsenal of products to assist the body's defense mechanisms that nature has so generously endowed us with. In this final chapter, I offer you a few hints for preparing your home for unexpected illnesses, ailments, and accidents. I hope you find this, as well as all you've learned so far, helpful in protecting yourself and your loved ones safely and naturally from the common irritations that come with living an active life.

Stocking Your Natural Medicine Cabinet

Preparing your home for unexpected emergencies is an important activity and should be planned carefully. The types of products you need to concern yourself with fall into two categories. The first category concerns products for common ailments and injuries. Every medicine cabinet should be stocked with products to remedy these unexpected emergencies. The second category concerns products for individual problems. For instance, everyone should have a natural product for cuts or burns, and something for an upset stomach. But a PMS formula would not be appropriate if you are a single man living alone, and there is no need for a teething remedy if there are no babies in the house. If you suffer from hay fever, you may choose to keep a natural hay fever product in your medicine chest, but it is not necessary for everyone to stock such a product.

I feel I can offer some guidelines for the first category, which will help you choose products that will fill general needs. That is what this chapter will basically try to cover. On the other hand, the second, more specific category of products you will have to evaluate for yourself. So, I will help you select a basic array of natural remedies for your home medicine cabinet, and you can add to this according to your individual needs. As you consider additional products, consider every member of your household as to their individual needs. At the end of this book is a product listing summarized for your convenience. Skim through this list to see if any of the products relate to the individual needs of you and your family. If they do, add them to the example of a basic product mix that I will show you now. Remember, this is only an example, as under some of the headings listed below there is the possibility of other choices.

- *Burns and cuts:*
  - ☐ **Hyland's Calendula Off. Tincture**
  - ☐ **Autumn Harp Comfrey Salve**

- *Constipation and diarrhea:*
  - ☐ **Nature's Way Cascara Sagrada** *or* **Nature's Herbs Cascara Sagrada** *or* **Energy Medicine Constipation**
  - ☐ **Energy Medicine Diarrhea**

- *Digestive problems:*
  - ☐ **Power Herbs Digest-Ease** *or* **Zand Digest Herbal Formula**
  - ☐ **Energy Medicine Nausea (Vomiting)**

- *Eye problems:*
  - ☐ **Similasan Eye Drops #1** *or* **Similasan Eye Drops #2**

- *Flu and cold care:*
  - ☐ **Energy Medicine Flu Solution** *or* **Oscillococcinum** *or* **Boericke & Tafel Alpha CF**
  - ☐ **Zand Insure Herbal** *or* **Yerba Prima Echinace**
  - ☐ **Energy Medicine Influenza/cold**
  - ☐ **Naturade Expec II**

- *Headache:*
  - ☐ **Power Herbs Willowprin**
  - ☐ **Nature's Herbs Dong Quai** (Also good for tight muscles.)

- *Insomnia:*
  - ☐ **Nature's Way Naturest** *or* **Yerba Prima Valerian Root**

- *Muscle sprains, spasms, and bruises:*
  - ☐ **Hyland's Arnica Lotion**

- *Sinus problems:*
  - ☐ **Nature's Cold Care**
  - ☐ **Power Herbs Bronc-ease**
  - ☐ **Breh Respiratory Rescue**

- *Sore throat:*
  - ☐ **Camocare Throat Spray/Gargle**

- ☐ **Zand HerbaLozenge Vitamin C Orange** *or* **Naturade Expec III Throat Lozenges**

- *Stress and emotional problems:*
  - ☐ **Yerba Prima Adaptoplex**
  - ☐ **Bach Rescue Remedy**
  - ☐ **Breh Calm Seas** (Also good for sore muscles, flu, and colds.)

So now you have some guidelines to outfit your medicine cabinet. You are ready to safely prepare your home for many unfortunate occurrences that can, from time to time, plague us and our loved ones. With fine products as healing partners, and a good balanced diet of nutritious natural foods, you are able to supplement the powerful defending mechanisms that nature has provided us with. Let's hope you never have to use them, but at least you can rest assured that you are ready and prepared to deal with the unexpected.

When You're on the Move!

You also may want to adapt this list for a first-aid kit when going camping, hiking, fishing, or traveling. Sometimes homeopathic products are especially helpful when traveling because they are usually in small containers. Because of their compact size, several remedies can be placed in a pack or suitcase without taking up too much space. Some suggestions for products you may want to consider for a first-aid kit are listed below. Again, you may want to adapt or add to this depending on the type of activity or according to special needs of you or your family members (i.e., if someone suffers from hay fever, etc.).

- *Burns, cuts, skin irritations, bites, and stings:*
  - [ ] **Hyland's Calendula Off. 1X Ointment** *or* **Autumn Harp Comfrey Salve**
  - [ ] **Breezy Balms Oak Away** (Also good for bites and stings.)
  - [ ] **Naturade Aloe Vera 80**
  - [ ] **Desert Essence Jojoba-Aloe Vera Lip Balm**

- *Constipation and diarrhea:*
  - [ ] **Energy Medicine Constipation**
  - [ ] **Energy Medicine Diarrhea**

- *Digestive problems:*
  - [ ] **Power Herbs Digest-Ease** *or* **Zand Digest Herbal Formula**
  - [ ] **Energy Medicine Nausea (Vomiting)**

- *Eye discomfort:*
  - [ ] **Similasan Eye Drops #1**

- *Flu and cold care:*
  - [ ] **Energy Medicine Flu Solution** *or* **Oscillococcinum** *or* **Boericke & Tafel Alpha CF**
  - [ ] **Energy Medicine Influenza/Cold**
  - [ ] **Zand HerbaLozenge Vitamin C Orange** *or* **Naturade Expec III Throat Lozenges**

- *Headache:*
  - [ ] **Power Herbs Willowprin** *or* **Energy Medicine Headache** *and* **Energy Medicine Headache/Neuralgia**

- *Muscle sprains, spasms, bruises, and fatigue:*
  - [ ] **Hyland's Arnica Lotion** (Don't forget cotton balls.)
  - [ ] **Energy Medicine Rheumatism** *and* **Muscle Fatigue**

- *Sinus problems:*
  - [ ] **Energy Medicine Sinus**

- *Stress, fright, and emotional problems:*
  - [ ] **Bach Rescue Remedy**

I hope that while reading this text you gained a better understanding of the human body and its remarkable abilities to preserve our health. I hope your appreciation grew, even just a little, for the complexity of life itself and the achievements of that awesome force that some call nature. Whatever you call it, you can't help but be impressed by its uncanny intelligence in the creation and maintenance of the network of systems that make up the living being. And I hope you have learned a few tricks to help you assist nature in accomplishing its ongoing goals.

I also hope this educational process, whether it is just beginning for you or an ongoing subject of study, will continue to grow. Our health is perhaps our most precious asset, for, without it, our existence can become extremely uncomfortable and our actions to some extent limited, not to mention the effect ill health can have on the length of our lives. The more we can learn about keeping our bodies healthy, the more we can enjoy and experience the beauty available to us without distraction.

Closing Thoughts

For yourself, treat your life with the respect it has so profoundly earned. Be informed and enjoy all this life has to offer, knowing clearly when your body needs proper attention and how to give that attention in a safe and conscious way. And remember, don't get so very serious about it that you create stress and cease having fun, for that is an illness as well.

If you are having difficulty locating any of the products mentioned in this book, write to me at Healing Partners, P.O. Box 547, Louisville, CO 80027. So for now, good-bye, and I sincerely hope you live a very long, healthy, and happy life.

References

Preface

1. Adams, J., "Cosmo's Guide to Alternative Medicine." *Cosmopolitan*, March 1986.

Chapter 1

1. Lebowitz, M., *Body Mechanics*. (MMI Press: New Hampshire), 1984, p. 102.
2. "Surgeon General's Report Is Healthy News for Natural Food." *Natural Foods Merchandiser*. October 1988, p. 4.
3. Mendelsohn, R. S., *How to Raise A Healthy Child . . . In Spite of Your Doctor*. (Ballantine Books: New York), 1984, p. 3.
4. Donsbach, K., *Drugs, Drugs and More Drugs*. (The International Institute of Natural Health Sciences: California), 1985, p. 18.
5. Ibid., p. 19.
6. Ibid., p. 19.
7. Ibid., p. 17.
8. Ibid., p. 1.

Chapter 2

1. Kaptchuk, T., "Tracing The Roots of Modern Herbalism." *Natural Foods Merchandiser*, October 1988.
2. "Is Herb Standardization Medicine For The Industry." *Natural Foods Merchandiser*. October 1989, p. 41.
3. Panos, M. and Heimlich, J., *Homeopathic Medicine At Home*. (J. P. Tarcher: New York), 1980.
4. Smith, D., *The Home Prescriber*. (Ehrhart & Karl: Chicago), 1964, p. 5.
5. Craig, C., *Homeopathy, What It Is And How It Works*. (Cecil Craig: Los Angeles), 1974, p. 4.
6. Lucas, R., *Nature's Medicines*. (Wilshire Book Co.: California), 1968, p. 20.
7. Edmunds, H. T., et al., *Some Unrecognized Factors In Medicine*. (The Theosophical Publishing House: Illinois), 1976, p. 125.
8. Ibid., p. 126.
9. Maltz, M., *Psycho-Cybernetics*. (Simon & Schuster: New York), 1960, p. 37.

10. Hay, L. L., *Heal Your Body*. (Coleman Publishing: New York), 1982, p. 1.

11. Thomas, S., *Massage For Common Ailments*. (Simon & Schuster: New York), 1989, p. 21.

12. *The Holistic Health Handbook*. (Berkeley Holistic Health Center: California), 1979, p. 15.

13. Ibid., p. 18.

Chapter 3

1. Finnegan, J., *Addictions, A Nutritional Approach to Recovery*. (Elysian Arts: California), 1988, p. 10.

2. Winter, R., *A Consumer's Dictionary Of Food Additives*. (Crown Publishers: New York), 1974, p. 2-3.

3. Cituk, K., and Finnegan, J., *Natural Foods And Good Cooking*. (Elysian Arts: California), 1989, p. 7.

4. Winter, *A Consumer's Dictionary Of Food Additives*, p. 2.

5. *Chemical Cuisine*. (Center For Science In The Public Interest: Washington, D.C.) 1985, p. 1.

6. Ibid., p. 1.

7. Winter, *A Consumer's Dictionary Of Food Additives*, p. 155.

8. Krizmanic, J., "What's in a Label?" *Vegetarian Times*, July 1989.

9. Levy, P., *More On Sugar And How It Gets That Way*. (Progenius Products: Massachusetts), 1980, p. 1.

10. Ibid., p. 3.

11. Ibid., p. 3.

12. Finnegan, *Addictions, A Nutritional Approach To Recovery*, p. 18.

13. Heller, L., *A Dietary Analysis Interpretation Guide*. (Heller: Colorado), 1984, p. 1.

14. Cituk and Finnegan, *Natural Foods And Good Cooking*, p. 15.

15. Ibid., p. 16.

16. Ronsard, N., *Cellulite: Those Lumps, Bumps, and Bulges You Couldn't Lose Before*. (Bantam Books: New York), 1975, p. 43.

17. Ibid., p. 45.

18. Sperling, D., "Cholesterol Levels Too High In Some Adults." *USA Today*, July 7, 1989, p. 1.

19. *The Oil Press, No. 2*. (Spectrum Marketing, Inc.: California), 1988, p. 5.

20. Ibid., p. 5.

21. Ibid., p. 5.

22. Winter, *A Consumer's Dictionary Of Food Additives*, p. 122.

23. Finnegan, J., "Getting To The Facts About Fats." excerpted from *Understanding Oils and Fats*, (Elysian Arts: California), 1989, p. 1.

24. Ibid., p. 2.

25. Gittleman, A. with Desgrey, J., *Beyond Pritikin*. (Bantam Books: New York), 1989, p. 30.

26. *Monounsaturated Vegetable Oils For Balanced Cholesterol*. (Spectrum Marketing, Inc.: California), 1988.

27. Ibid.

28. Patrick, J., *Lowered Blood Pressure Linked To Heart Attacks*. (Alacer Corp.: California), 1989.

29. Donsbach, K., *The Donlsbach Report*. (Donsbach: California), January, 1989, vol. 1, no. 1, p. 9.

30. Airola, P., *Are You Confused*. (Health Plus Publishers: Arizona), 1976.

31. Patrick, *Lowered Blood Pressure Linked To Heart Attacks*.

32. "Hypertension Update," *Prevention*, January 1989, vol. 41, no. 1.

33. Patrick, *Lowered Blood Pressure Linked To Heart Attacks*.

34. Ibid.

35. "Hypertension Update," *Prevention*.

36. Airola, *Are You Confused*.

37. Heller, *A Dietary Analysis Interpretation Guide*, p. 1.

38. Berry, L., *Internal Cleansing*. (Bontanica Press: California), 1985, p. 29.

39. Cituk and Finnegan, *Natural Foods and Good Cooking*, p. 21.

40. Berry, *Internal Cleansing*, p. 43.

41. Grey, R., *The Colon Health Handbook*. (Emerald Publishing: Nevada), 1985, p. 41.

42. *Yesterday, Today, and Tomorrow*. (NBC TV: New York), August 2, 1989.

43. *Whole Foods Natural Foods Guide*. (Whole Foods Publishing: California), 1979, p. 31.

44. Ibid., p. 31.

45. Ibid., p. 31–32.

46. Dittmar, M., "Positively Speaking, The American Food Supply: How Safe Is Safe? Part IV." *Health Foods Business*, (Howmark Publishing: New Jersey), September, 1989, vol. 35, no. 9, p. 15.

47. Ibid., p. 15.

48. "A" Is For Apples. *60 Minutes*, (CBS News: New York), February 26, 1989, p. 10.

49. Ibid., p. 11.

50. "Bad Apples." *Consumer's Report*, May 1989.

51. "Dining With Invisible Danger." *Time Magazine*, March 27, 1989.

52. "How Safe Is Your Food." *Newsweek*, March 27, 1989.

53. Ibid.

54. "Dining With Invisible Danger." *Time Magazine*.

55. "A" Is For Apples. *60 Minutes*, p. 12,13.

56. Baily, C., *Fit Or Fat*. (Houghton Mifflin Company: Massachusetts), 1978, p. 24.

57. Ibid., p. 25.

58. Airola, *Are You Confused*.

59. Berry, *Internal Cleansing*, p. 47.

Chapter 4

1. "On Lysine Herbal." *Zand Herbal Notes*, (McZand Herbal: California) 1989.

2. Ibid.

3. Bricklin, M., *The Practical Encyclopedia Of Natural Healing*. (Rodale Press: Pennsylvania), 1976, p. 93.

4. *Fiberdophilus Information Sheet*. (Yerba Prima: California), 1989.

5. Kilmartin, A., *Cystitis, The Complete Self-Help Guide*. (Warner Books: California), 1980.

6. Bricklin, *The Practical Encyclopedia Of Natural Healing*, p. 94.

7. *An Interview With Dr. Howell On The Value Of Food Enzymes*. (Food Enzyme Research Foundation: Florida), 1979, p. 2.

8. Ibid.

9. Santillo, H., *Food Enzymes, The Missing Link To Radiant Health*. (Hohm Press: Arizona), 1987, p. 14.

10. Ibid., p. 22.

11. Howell, E., *Enzyme Nutrition, The Food Enzyme Concept*. (Avery Publishing Group: New Jersey), 1985, p. 29.

12. *The Zand Formulas, Product Information*. (McZand Herbal: California), 1989.

13. *Power Herbs Digest Ease*. (Nature's Herbs: Utah), 1987, (label).

14. *Nature's Remedy For Indigestion*. (Miracle Exclusives: California), 1989.

15. *Foundation Enzymes, The Missing Link To Radiant Health*. (Rainbow Light Nutritional Systems: California), 1989.

16. *An Interview With Dr. Howell On The Value Of Food Enzymes*, p. 7.

17. Ibid., p. 7.

18. Blitz, J. J., Smith, J. W., and Gerard, J. R., "Peptic Ulcer Therapy By Aloe Vera Gel, A Preliminary Report." *Journal of the American Osteopathic Association*, April, 1963, vol. 62.

19. Ibid.

20. Bricklin, *The Practical Encyclopedia Of Natural Healing*, p. 506.

21. Berry, *Internal Cleansing*, p. 49.

22. Lebowitz, *Body Mechanics*, p. 89.

23. Grey, *The Colon Health Handbook*, p. 6.

24. Lebowitz, *Body Mechanics*, p. 89–90.

25. Plant, M., *The Doctor's Guide To You And Your Colon*. (Harper & Row: New York), 1982.

26. Jackson M., and Terri Teague, *The Handbook of Alternatives To Chemical Medicine*. (Lawton-Teague Publications: California), 1975, p. 53.

27. Christopher, J., *School Of Natural Healing*. (Microlith Printing: Utah), 1976, p. 175.

28. Ibid., p. 175.

29. Bland, J., *Intestinal Toxicity And Inner Cleansing*. (Keats Publishing: Connecticut), 1987, p. 12.

30. Bricklin, *The Practical Encyclopedia Of Natural Healing*, p. 139.

31. Lebowitz, *Body Mechanics*, p. 92.

32. *Nature's Way Products, Natural Laxatives*. (Nature's Way Products: Utah), 1988.

33. Bland, J., and Cain, S., *Clinical Study of Yerba Prima Internal Cleansing Program In Human Subjects*. (Linus Pauling Institute Of Science And Medicine: California), 1988, p. 3.

34. "New Evidence Of Calcium." *The Herbalist*, (Yerba Prima Botanicals: California), Fall, 1989, p. 1.

35. Slattery, M., "Dietary Calcium Intake As A Mitigation Factor In Colon Cancer." *American Journal of Epidemiology*, 1988, vol. 128.

36. Lebowitz, *Body Mechanics*, p. 62.

37. Fintelmann, V., "Toxic Metabolic Hepatic Dysfunction And Its Management." *Aeitschrift Fur Phytotherapie*, 1986, p. 65.

38. "Milk Thistle: A Living Legend." *Whole Foods*, April, 1988, p. 79.

39. Salmi, H., and Sarna, S., "Effects Of Silymarin On Chemical, Functional and Morphological Alterations Of The Liver, A Double-Blind Controlled Study." *Scandinavian Journal of Gastroenterology*, 1982, p. 517.

40. Ibid., p. 517.
41. "Milk Thistle: A Living Legend." *Whole Foods*, p. 79.
42. Fintelmann, V., "Toxic Metabolic Hepatic Dysfunction And Its Management." *Zeitschrift Fur Phytotherapie*, p. 65.
43. "Detoxification Using Aged Garlic Extract." *The Health Professional*, (International Health Promotions: Lane Cove, NSW), 1988, p. 3.
44. Ibid., p. 3.
45. Santillo, *Food Enzymes, The Missing Link To Radiant Health*, p. 31.
46. Ibid., p. 7.
47. *American Journal Of Digestive Diseases, 5.* 1988. p. 184–9.
48. Kulvinskas, V., *Survival Into The 21st Century.* (Omangod Press: Iowa), 1975, p. 22.

Chapter 5

1. Jacob, S. W. and Francone, C. A., *Elements of Anatomy and Physiology.* (W. B. Saunders Co: Pennsylvania), 1976, p. 131.
2. Ibid., p. 136.
3. Zand, J., "Talking About Health." *Lifelines.* Summer, 1989, vol. 1, no. 1.
4. "Supplementary Strategies For A Winning Winter Season." *Delicious.* (New Hope Publications: Pennsylvania), November/December, 1986, p. 7.
5. Ibid., p. 7.
6. Fox, A., and Fox, B., "Keeping Your Immune System Strong." *Let's Live*, (T. K. Vodrey: California), August, 1989, p. 28.
7. Ibid., p. 30.
8. Ibid., p. 31.
9. *International Medical Statistics Survey.* (based on units sold) December 30, 1984.
10. Lampe, F., "Confirmation Of Homeopathy." *Natural Foods Merchandiser*, (New Hope Publications: Colorado), October, 1989, p. 32.
11. *Oscillococcinum, Important Facts And Merchandising Tips.* (Boiron Laboratories: Pennsylvania), 1985.
12. *Alpha CF For Colds & Flu.* (Boericke & Tafel: Pennsylvania), 1989.
13. Ibid.
14. Chone, B., "Ceziete Steuerung Der Leukozytentinetik Durch Echinacin." *Arzneimittel-Forshung* 1985.
15. Semachowiez, E., Urbandka, L., Manka, W., and Stolarska, E., "Evaluation of the Effect of Calendula Officinalis and Echinacea Augustifolia On Extracts On Trichomonusvaginalis In Vitro." *Wiadomosci Parazytolohiczne*, 1979.
16. Mowrey, D., *The Scientific Validation Of Herbs.* (Cormorant Books: USA), 1986, p. 119.
17. Ibid., p. 118.
18. Schimel, K., and Werner, G., "Nonspecific Enhancement of Intrinsic Resistance to Infection by Echinacin." *Ther. D. Gegenw*, 1981, p. 1065.
19. Ibid., p. 1065.
20. Mowrey, *The Scientific Validation of Herbs*, p. 158.
21. Badgley, L., "Strengthen Your Immune System With Natural Therapies." *Health World*, (Health World: California), September/October, 1988, p. 10.

22. Zand, J., "A Note From Dr. Zand." *Zand Herbal Talk, Vol. 2, No. 3* (McZand Herbal: California), 1988, p. 1.

23. Mowrey, *The Scientific Validation Of Herbs*, p. 122.

24. *Garlic, Garlicin.* (Nature's Way: Utah) 1988, p. 1.

25. Cavallito, C. and Baily, J., "Allicin, The Antibacterial Principle Of Allium Sativum. I. Isolation, Physical Properties and Antibacterial Action." *Journal of the American Chemical Society*, 1945, p. 1950-1951.

26. "Garlic In Cryptococcal Meningitis, A Preliminary Report Of 21 Cases." *Chinese Medical Journal*, (Hunan Medical College: China), 1980.

27. Bogacki, A., *Raw Garlic Can Cause Injury.* November 17, 1989.

28. Cavallito, and Baily, "Allicin, The Antibacterial Principle Of Allium Sativum. I. Isolation, Physical Properties and Antibacterial Action." *Journal of the American Chemical Society*, p. 1950.

29. *Garlic, Garlicin*, p. 1.

30. Brewer, W., *Odorless, Aged Garlic For Unexcelled Benefits.* (excerpt provided by Wakanaga of America), p. 1.

31. Sumiyoshi, D. H., *Some Unique Benefits Of Kyolic.* (Wakunaga of America: California), 1989, p. 2.

32. Lau, B., *Garlic For Health.* (Lotus Light Publications: Wisconsin), 1988, p. 8.

33. Brewer, *Odorless, Aged Garlic For Unexcelled Benefits*, p. 3.

34. Ibid., p. 3.

35. Bogacki, *Raw Garlic Can Cause Injury.*

36. Brewer, W., *Questions on Garlic.* December 26, 1989.

37. Bogacki, *Raw Garlic Can Cause Injury.*

38. *Tis The Season.* (Makers of Kal: California), 1989.

39. Patrick, J., *What Vitamin C Can Do For You, "The Super Carbo."* (Alacer Corporation: California), 1989.

40. Ibid.

41. Armes, C., *Botanical Sea Bath Creations, Introducing; The Luxury Bath With Multiple Health Benefits.* (Breh Laboratories: Colorado), 1989.

42. *The Zand Formulas, Product Information*, p. 1.

43. *Medicine From Nature.* (Nature's Way Products: Utah), 1988.

44. *Natural Health Care For Everybody.* (Naturpharma: California), 1987.

45. Tortora, G. J., and Anagnostakos, N. P., *Principles Of Anatomy And Physiology.* (Harper & Row: New York) 1987, p. 144.

46. Ibid., p. 144.

47. *Tis The Season.*

48. *Allerin.* (Healthcare Naturals: Utah) 1987.

49. *Notes On The Zand Product Line.* (McZand Herbal: California), 1989.

50. *Medicine From Nature.*

51. Wiesenauer, M., Haussler, S., and Gaus, W., "Pollinosis Therapy With Galphimia Glauca." *Fortschritte Der Therapie.* (excerpts provided by Bioforce USA).

52. *Hayfever.* (Longevity Pure Medicine: California), 1986. (label)

53. *Allergy Relief.* (BioAllers: Washington), 1989.

54. *Notes On The Zand Product Line.*

55. Lau, *Garlic For Health*, p. 29.

56. *Food Sensitivity System.* (Rainbow Light Nutritional Systems: California), 1989, p. 2.

57. Ibid., p. 2.

58. Ibid., p. 3.

59. *Allergy Relief.*
60. Astor, S., M.D., *Hidden Food Allergies.* (Avery Publishing Group: New York), 1986, p. 6.

Chapter 6

1. Jacob and Francone, *Elements of Anatomy and Physiology,* p. 177.
2. Bricklin, *The Practical Encyclopedia Of Natural Healing,* p. 182.
3. Mowrey, *The Scientific Validation Of Herbs,* p. 224.
4. *Feverfew Information Sheet.* (Yerba Prima Botanicals: California), 1989.
5. "New Feverfew Headache Research." *Herbalgram, No. 18/19,* (Herb Research Foundation and The American Herbal Products Association: California) Fall/Winter, 1989, p. 6.
6. *Feverfew.* (Nature's Way Products: Utah) 1987.
7. Hoffman, D., "Your Herbal Home Medicine Chest." *The Self Care Health Library.* (Keats Publishing: Connecticut) 1989, p. 23.
8. Tyler, R., *The Honest Herbal.* 1981.
9. *Adaptoplex Adaptogen Formula.* (Yerba Prima Botanicals: California), 1987, p. 2.
10. Ibid., p. 4.
11. Ibid., p. 4.
12. Vlamis, G., "Bach Flower Remedy, Homeopathy In The Home." *Homeopathy Today, Vol. II, No. 8,* (Ellon Bach USA: New York), 1982, p. 1.
13. Ibid., p. 1
14. *Hyland's Home Remedies.* (Standard Homeopathic Company: California), 1989, p. 2.
15. Lau, *Garlic For Health,* p. 56.
16. Cochun, J., *Rainbow Light Nutritional Systems.* (Rainbow Light Nutritional Systems: California), 1988.
17. *Similasan Eyedrops #1, Swiss Homeopathic Remedy.* (Similasan Corporation: Washington), 1989.
18. *Similasan Eyedrops #2, Swiss Homeopathic Remedy.* (Similasan Corporation: Washington), 1989.
19. *Similasan Homeopathic Remedies, You'll Feel Better Without Chemicals.* (Similasan Corporation: Washington), 1989.
20. Dransfield, C., *Beating Jet Lag.* (Quantas Airlines: Australia), 1989.
21. Vlamis, "Bach Flower Remedy, Homeopathy In The Home," *Homeopathy Today, Vol. II, No. 8,* p. 1.
22. *Motion Sickness.* (Nature's Way Products: Utah) 1987.
23. Mowrey, *The Scientific Validation Of Herbs,* p. 164.
24. Bricklin, *The Practical Encyclopedia Of Natural Healing,* p. 300.
25. Mowrey, *The Scientific Validation Of Herbs,* p. 215.
26. *Product Information.* (Yerba Prima Botanicals: California), 1989.
27. *Journal Of Natural Products,* 43:721. November/December, 1980.
28. *Hyland's Home Remedies,* p. 2.
29. Bricklin, *The Practical Encyclopedia Of Natural Healing,* p. 301.
30. Baranowski, Z., *Stress And Free Radicals.* 1988.
31. Wagner, E., *The Gift Of The Ancients, Ginkgo Biloba.* (Nutrition Institute Publishing Company: Indiana), p. 2.
32. Ibid., p. 4.
33. *Nutrimental, Ginkgo Biloba.* (Yerba Prima Botanicals: California), 1987.

34. Schuitemaker, G., "Ginkgo Against Senility." *Ortho Supplement NR.* 2, 1988.

35. Ibid.

Chapter 7

1. Jacob and Francone, *Elements of Anatomy and Physiology*, p. 106.
2. Lebowitz, *Body Mechanics*, p. 112.
3. Ibid., p. 113.
4. Ibid., p. 113.
5. Ibid., p. 114.
6. Fox, A., M.D., and Fox, B., Ph.D., "Conquering Hypertension—The Silent Killer." *Let's Live Magazine*, (T. K. Vodrey, California), May, 1989, p. 26.
7. Gittleman and Desgrey, *Beyond Pritikin*, p. 33.
8. Ibid., p. 18.
9. Lebowitz, *Body Mechanics*, p. 114.
10. Bland, J., "Subjects Of The Heart." *Delicious Magazine*, (New Hope Publications: Pennsylvania), vol. 5, no. 3, April, 1989, p. 7.
11. Ibid., p. 7.
12. Patrick, J., *Lowered Blood Pressure Linked To Heart Attacks*, p. 1.
13. Gittleman and Desgrey, *Beyond Pritikin*, p. 42–43.
14. Ibid., p. 44.
15. Bland, "Subjects Of The Heart," p. 8.
16. "Facts About Rice." *Natural Velocity News.* (Natural Gourmet Foods: Illinois), July/August, 1989.
17. Lebowitz, *Body Mechanics*, p. 115.
18. Patrick, J., *Lowered Blood Pressure Linked To Heart Attacks*, p. 1.
19. Ibid., p. 1.
20. Ibid., p. 1.
21. Ibid., p. 1.
22. Moore and Webb, *The K Factor.*
23. Patrick, J., *Lowered Blood Pressure Linked To Heart Attacks*, p. 1.
24. Lebowitz, *Body Mechanics*, p. 115.
25. Bland, "Subjects Of The Heart," p. 7.
26. "Nature's Way." *America's Natural Healthcare Catalog*, (Nature's Way Products: Utah), 1988, p. 26.
27. Ibid., p. 26.
28. Lau, *Garlic For Health*, p. 25–26.
29. *A Review Of The Benefits Of Garlic.* (Wakunaga Of America: California), 1989.
30. Jackson and Teague, *The Handbook Of Alternatives To Chemical Medicine*, p. 84.
31. Donsbach, *The Donsbach Report, Vol. 1, No. 1*, p. 3.
32. Wagner, *The Gift Of The Ancients, Ginkgo Biloba*, p. 7.
33. *Nutrimental, Ginkgo Biloba.* (Yerba Prima Botanicals: California), 1987.
34. Bricklin, *The Practical Encyclopedia Of Natural Healing*, p. 521.
35. Ibid., p. 521.
36. Ibid., p. 521.
37. Ibid., p. 522.
38. *Hyland's Hemmorex Hemorrhoids.* (Standard Homeopathic Company: California), 1989. (label)

Chapter 8

1. *Nature's Way, Premenstrual Syndrome, Efamol PMS.* (Nature's Way Products: Utah), 1987.
2. "On PMS Herbal. *Zand Herbal Notes,* (McZand Herbal: California), 1989.
3. *Nature's Way, Premenstrual Syndrome, Efamol PMS.* (label)
4. Ibid.
5. Ibid.
6. Ibid.
7. Snyder, T., "Women's Health Products Require Knowledge, Service." *Natural Foods Merchandiser,* (New Hope Publications: Colorado), December, 1989, p. 21.
8. Zimmerman, P., "Pre-menstrual And Pre-Natal Nutrition." *Health World, Vol. 2, No. 6,* (Health World Inc: California), p. 26.
9. "On PMS Herbal. *Zand Herbal Notes.*
10. Abraham and Hargrove, *Effect Of Vitamin B6. . . . Infertility.* 1980.
11. Zimmerman, "Pre-menstrual And Pre-Natal Nutrition." *Health World,* p. 26.
12. Abraham, "Primary Dysmenorrhea." *Clinical Obstetrics and Gynecology,* 1985.
13. Zimmerman, "Pre-menstrual And Pre-Natal Nutrition." *Health World,* p. 26.
14. Finnegan, J., *Regeneration Of Health.* (Elysian Arts: California), 1987, p. 34–35.
15. "Nature's Way." *America's Natural Healthcare Catalog,* p. 26.
16. Guiltinan, J., "The Natural Pharmacy, Stocking The Medicine Chest." *Health Foods Business,* (Howmark Publishing: New Jersey), July, 1989, p. 42.
17. Huges, "A New Look At Dietary Fiber." *Human Nutrition, Clinical Nutrition,* 1985.
18. Lebowitz, *Body Mechanics,* p. 109.
19. *Homeopathic Reference Manual.* (Natra-Bio: Washington), 1989, p. 522.
20. Bricklin, *The Practical Encyclopedia Of Natural Healing,* p. 535.
21. *The Candida Combo D-Yeast And Nutra-Mune.* (Parametric Associates: Missouri), 1989.
22. Bricklin, *The Practical Encyclopedia Of Natural Healing,* p. 536.
23. Ibid., p. 536.
24. *Caprinex And Sodium Caprylate: Your Customer's Questions Answered.* (Nature's Way Products: Utah), 1988.
25. *Micro-Flora Highlights.* (Micro-Flora Corporation: California) 1989.
26. "Menopause Hormone Linked To Increased Cancer Threat, Combination Of Estrogen, Progestin Assessed." *The Denver Post/National,* (from *The New York Times*) Thursday, August 3, 1989, p. 4a.
27. *The Herbal Male Toning System.* (Rainbow Light Nutritional Systems: California), 1988.
28. Mowrey, *The Scientific Validation Of Herbs,* p. 287.
29. "Chinese Ginseng Root, Standardized Extract (Panax Ginseng)." *Yerba Prima, Herbs To Live By, Product Information,* (Yerba Prima Botanicals: California), 1989.

30. "Siberian Ginseng Root, Eleutherococcus Senticosus, Prima Standardized Extract, 0.2% Eleutheroside E." *Yerba Prima, Herbs To Live By*, (Yerba Prima Botanicals: California), 1989.
31. Malstrom, S., N.D., M. T., "Ginseng—A Many Varied Herb." *Dial Herbs Newsletter*, (Dial Herbs: Utah), April 1989, p. 3.
32. "Siberian Ginseng Root, Eleutherococcus Senticosus, Prima Standardized Extract, 0.2% Eleutheroside E." *Yerba Prima, Herbs To Live By*.
33. Malstrom, "Ginseng—A Many Varied Herb." *Dial Herbs Newsletter*, p. 3.
34. Ibid., p. 3.
35. "Siberian Ginseng Root, Eleutherococcus Senticosus, Prima Standardized Extract, 0.2% Eleutheroside E." *Yerba Prima, Herbs To Live By*.
36. *Zand Herbal Talk, Quarterly Newsletter, Vol. 3, No. 3.* (McZand Herbal: California), Fall, 1989, p. 2.
37. Ibid., p. 2.
38. *The Herbal Male Toning System.* p. 2.
39. Mowrey, *The Scientific Validation Of Herbs*, p. 88–89.
40. *Zand Herbal Formulas.* (McZand Herbal: California), 1989.
41. Null, G. et al., *The Complete Question & Answer Book Of Natural Therapy.* (Dell Publishing: New York) 1972, p. 90–91.
42. Ibid., p. 92.
43. Bricklin, *The Practical Encyclopedia Of Natural Healing*, p. 427.
44. Ibid., p. 427.
45. Jonsson, G., *Swedish Medical Journal.* (58:2487) 1961.
46. Bricklin, *The Practical Encyclopedia Of Natural Healing*, p. 427.
47. "Nature's Way Nutritional Supplement, Bee Pollen." *America's Natural Healthcare Company*, (Nature's Way Products: Utah) 1986.

Chapter 9

1. Jacob and Francone, *Elements of Anatomy and Physiology*, p. 34.
2. Tortora and Anagnostakos, *Principles Of Anatomy And Physiology*, p. 192.
3. Ibid., p. 212.
4. Tyler, *The Honest Herbal*, 1981.
5. *Camocare Combines Science With Nature.* (Abkit, Inc: New York), 1988.
6. Ibid.
7. Tortora and Anagnostakos, *Principles Of Anatomy And Physiology*, p. 191.
8. Hoffman, "Your Herbal Home Medicine Chest." *The Self Care Health Library*, p. 20–21.
9. The American National Red Cross, *First Aid, Fourth Edition.* (Doubleday & Company: New York), 1965, p. 71.
10. Shepherd, D., *Homeopathy For The First-Aider.* (Health Science Press: Sussex, England), 1972, p. 26.
11. *Fresh Comfrey Salve With Goldenseal.* (Autumn Harp: Vermont), 1989.
12. Ibid.
13. *The Finest Name In Tree Tea Oils.* (Dessert Essence: California), 1989.
14. *Sssstingstop Soothing Gel.* (Boericke & Tafel: Pennsylvania), 1989.
15. "Insect Bites." *Natra-Bio Homeopathic Reference Manual*, Natra-Bio: Washington), 1989, p. 535.

Chapter 10

    1. Mendelsohn, *How to Raise A Healthy Child . . . In Spite of Your Doctor*, p. 10.

    2. Ibid., p. 37.

    3. Ibid., p. 52.

    4. Cituk and Finnegan, *Natural Foods and Good Cooking*, p. 18.

    5. Ibid., p. 18.

    6. Mendelsohn, *How to Raise A Healthy Child . . . In Spite of Your Doctor*, p. 3.

    7. Ibid., p. 3.

    8. Ibid., p. 3.

    9. *Be Prepared For Emergencies With Homeopathic Medicines For Children.* (P & S Laboratories: California), 1988, p. 3.

    10. Ibid., p. 3.

    11. Mendelsohn, *How to Raise A Healthy Child . . . In Spite of Your Doctor*, p. 175.

    12. *Hyland's Home Remedies*, p. 2.

Remedies at a Glance

Major physical problems and conditions are shown here with a list of appropriate natural remedies. For a fuller explanation on the properties and uses of these remedies, consult the specific chapters mentioned.

Allergies (*See Chapter 5*)

- [ ] bioAllers Allergy Relief: Animal Hair/Dander
- [ ] bioAllers Allergy Relief: Mold/Yeast/Dust
- [ ] bioAllers Allergy Relief: Pollen/Hayfever
- [ ] bioAllers Food Allergies: Dairy
- [ ] bioAllers Food Allergies: Grain
- [ ] Bioforce Pollinosan
- [ ] Kyolic Aged Garlic Extract
- [ ] Longevity Hayfever
- [ ] Nature's Herbs Allerin
- [ ] Nature's Way Allerex
- [ ] Nature's Way Broncrin
- [ ] Power Herbs Allerelief
- [ ] Rainbow Light Food Sensitivity System
- [ ] Similasan Eye Drops #2
- [ ] Zand Decongest Herbal Formula
- [ ] Zand Insure Herbal
  See also Hay fever.

Bites, Insect
(*See Skin Irritations*)

Bone Injuries (*See Chapter 9*)

- [ ] Hyland's Symphytum 12X

Burns and Cuts (*See Chapter 9*)

- [ ] Hyland's Calendula Off. Tincture
- [ ] Hyland's Calendula Off. 1X Ointment
- [ ] Hyland's Calendula Oil
- [ ] Naturade Aloe Vera 80

Cardiovascular Nutrition
(*See Chapter 7*)

- [ ] Alacer Super-Gram II
- [ ] Arrowhead Mills Fresh Flax Seed Oil
- [ ] Enzyme Complex-Kyolic Formula 102
- [ ] Nature's Way Efamol EPO

225

☐ Nature's Way Efamol
   Omega-3 Fish Oils (EPA)
☐ Nature's Way Garlicin
☐ Nature's Way North
   American Oat Fiber
☐ Nature's Way Red Clover
   Combination Formula
☐ Spectrum Naturals
   Veg-Omega-3
☐ Yerba Prima Adaptoplex

Children (*See Chapter 10*)

☐ Autumn Harp Comfrey
   Salve
☐ Bach Rescue Remedy
☐ Hyland's Bed Wetting
   Tablets
☐ Hyland's Calms
☐ Hyland's Colic Tablets
☐ Hyland's Cough Syrup
   with Honey
☐ Hyland's Teething Tablets
☐ Kyolic Aged Garlic Extract
☐ Nature's Way
   Primadophilus for
   Children
☐ Nature's Way
   Primadophilus Junior

Circulation (*See Chapter 7*)

☐ Nature's Way Ginkgold
☐ Yerba Prima Nutrimental

Colds and Flu (*See Chapter 5*)

☐ Alacer Corp. E-mergen-C
☐ Alacer Super-Gram II
☐ Boericke & Tafel Alpha CF
☐ Boiron Borneman
   Oscillococcinum
☐ Breh Botanical Sea Bath
   Creations

☐ Breh Perspir•detox
☐ Energy Medicine Flu
   Solution
☐ Energy Medicine
   Influenza/Cold
☐ Flora Laboratories
   Florammune Echinacea
☐ Kal LoZINCges
☐ Kyolic Aged Garlic Extract
☐ Nature's Way Garlicin
☐ Yerba Prima Echinace
☐ Zand Insure Herbal

Colon Cleansing (*See Chapter 4*)

☐ Yerba Prima Aloe Vera plus
   Herbs
☐ Yerba Prima Internal
   Cleansing Program:
   Yerba Prima Colon Care
   Formula *and*
   Yerba Prima Kalenite
☐ Yerba Prima Vivalo Creme

Colon Problems (*See Chapter 4*)

☐ Energy Medicine
   Constipation
☐ Energy Medicine Diarrhea
☐ Energy Medicine Nausea
   (Vomiting)
☐ Nature's Herbs Cascara
   Sagrada
☐ Nature's Way Fiber Cleanse
☐ Nature's Way Garlicin
☐ Nature's Way
   Primadophilus
☐ Yerba Prima Chamomile
☐ Yerba Prima Echinace
☐ Yerba Prima Fiberdophilus

Coughs (*See Sore Throats
and Coughs*)

Cuts (*See Burns*)

Eye Problems (*See Chapter 6*)

- ☐ Similasan Eye Drops #1
- ☐ Similasan Eye Drops #2

Female Problems (*See Chapter 8*)

- ☐ Living Source Complete B-Complex Nutrient System
- ☐ Flora Balance
- ☐ Natra-Bio Bladder Irritation
- ☐ Nature's Herbs Dong Quai
- ☐ Nature's Way Caprinex
- ☐ Nature's Way Primadophilus
- ☐ Nutrapathic D-Yeast
- ☐ Nutrapathic Nutra-Mune
- ☐ Yerba Prima Dong Quai
- ☐ Yerba Prima Fiberdophilus
  See also Menstrual Problems.

Flu (See *Colds and Flu*)

Hay Fever (*See Chapter 5*)

- ☐ bioAllers Allergy Relief: Pollen/Hayfever
- ☐ Bioforce Pollinosan
- ☐ Kyolic Aged Garlic Extract
- ☐ Longevity Hayfever
- ☐ Nature's Herbs Allerin
- ☐ Power Herbs Allerelief
- ☐ Similasan Eye Drops #2

Headaches (*See Chapter 6*)

- ☐ Energy Medicine Headache
- ☐ Medicine Headache/Neuralgia
- ☐ Nature's Herbs Dong Quai
- ☐ Power Herbs Willowprin

- ☐ Yerba Prima Dong Quai
- ☐ Yerba Prima Feverfew

Heart (*See Cardiovascular Nutrition*)

Hemorrhoids (*See Chapter 7*)

- ☐ Energy Medicine Hemorrhoids/Pile
- ☐ Hyland's Calendula Off. 1X Ointment
- ☐ Hyland's Calendula Oil
- ☐ Hyland's Hemmorex

Indigestion (*See Chapter 4*)

- ☐ Energy Medicine Nausea (Vomiting)
- ☐ Floradix Herbal Bitters
- ☐ Power Herbs Digest-Ease
- ☐ Rainbow Light All-Zyme
- ☐ Yerba Prima Aloe Vera plus Herbs
- ☐ Yerba Prima Chamomile
- ☐ Zand Digest Herbal Formula

Insomnia (*See Chapter 6*)

- ☐ Boiron Borneman Nervousness/Insomnia
- ☐ Hyland's Calms
- ☐ Nature's Way Naturest
- ☐ Yerba Prima Chamomile
- ☐ Yerba Prima Valerian Root

Liver Function (*See Chapter 4*)

- ☐ Floradix Herbal Bitters
- ☐ Kyolic Aged Garlic Extract
- ☐ Nature's Way Thisilyn
- ☐ Rainbow Light All-Zyme
- ☐ Yerba Prima LivCleanse

Male Problems (*See Chapter 8*)

- ☐ Nature's Way Bee Pollen
- ☐ Rainbow Light Male Toning System
- ☐ Yerba Prima Chinese Ginseng
- ☐ Yerba Prima Siberian Ginseng
- ☐ Zand Active Herbal
- ☐ Zand Male Formula

Memory (*See Chapter 6*)

- ☐ Breh Alert and Alive
- ☐ Nature's Way Ginkgold
- ☐ Yerba Prima Nutrimental

Menstrual Problems
(*See Chapter 8*)

- ☐ Nature's Way Change-O-Life Formula
- ☐ Nature's Way Efamol EPO
- ☐ Yerba Prima Colon Care Formula
- ☐ Zand Female Formula
- ☐ Zand PMS Herbal
  See also Female Problems.

Mouth Sores (*See Chapter 4*)

- ☐ Bach Rescue Remedy
- ☐ Energy Medicine Fever Blister or Canker Sore
- ☐ Hyland's Calendula Off. Tincture
- ☐ Nature's Way Primadophilus
- ☐ Yerba Prima Adaptoplex
- ☐ Yerba Prima Fiberdophilus
- ☐ Zand Lysine Herbal

Muscle Problems
(*See Chapter 9*)

- ☐ Breezy Balms Warm Up Rub
- ☐ Breh Athlete's Relief
- ☐ Breh Healthy Joints
- ☐ Camocare Pain Relieving Cream
- ☐ Energy Medicine Rheumatism and Muscle Fatigue
- ☐ Hyland's Arnica Lotion
- ☐ Longevity Arthritis Pain
- ☐ Nature's Herbs Dong Quai
- ☐ Yerba Prima Dong Quai

Nausea and Vomiting
(*See Chapter 4*)

- ☐ Energy Medicine Nausea (Vomiting)

Prostate Problems
(*See Chapter 8*)

- ☐ Nature's Way Bee Pollen

Senility (*See Memory*)

Sinus Congestion
(*See Chapter 5*)

- ☐ Autumn Harp Comfrey Salve
- ☐ Breezy Balms Warm Up Rub
- ☐ Breh Respiratory Rescue
- ☐ Energy Medicine Sinus
- ☐ Hyland's Calendula Off. 1X Ointment
- ☐ Nature's Way Nature's Cold Care
- ☐ Olbas Inhaler
- ☐ Power Herbs Bronc-ease
- ☐ Zand Decongest Herbal

Skin Irritations (*See Chapter 9*)

- [ ] Autumn Harp Comfrey Salve
- [ ] Boericke & Tafel Sssstingstop Soothing Gel
- [ ] Breezy Balms Oak Away
- [ ] Desert Essence Jojoba-Aloe Vera Lip Balm
- [ ] Hyland's Anacarium 3X
- [ ] Kangaroo Brand Australian Tea Tree Oil Lip Balm
- [ ] Natra-Bio Insect Bites

Sleep Problems (*See Insomnia*)

Sore Throats and Coughs (*See Chapter 5*)

- [ ] Breezy Balms Warm Up Rub
- [ ] Camocare Throat Spray/Gargle
- [ ] Kal LoZINCges
- [ ] Naturade Expec
- [ ] Naturade Expec II
- [ ] Naturade Expec III Throat Lozenges
- [ ] Power Herbs Bronc-ease
- [ ] Zand HerbaLozenge
- [ ] Zand HerbaLozenge Vitamin C Orange

Stings, Insect (*See Skin Irritations*)

Stress (*See Chapter 6*)

- [ ] Bach Rescue Remedy
- [ ] Breh Calm Seas
- [ ] Hyland's Calms
- [ ] Kyolic Aged Garlic Extract
- [ ] Living Source Complete B-Complex Nutrient System
- [ ] Similasan Eye Drops #1
- [ ] Similasan Eye Drops #2
- [ ] Yerba Prima Adaptoplex

Travel Sickness (*See Chapter 6*)

- [ ] Bach Rescue Remedy
- [ ] Hyland's Arnica 30X
- [ ] Power Herbs Travel-Ease
- [ ] Yerba Prima Adaptoplex

Ulcers (*See Chapter 4*)

- [ ] Hyland's Calms
- [ ] Yerba Prima Adaptoplex
- [ ] Yerba Prima Aloe Vera plus Herbs

Varicose Veins (*See Chapter 7*)

- [ ] Miracle Salve
- [ ] Nature's Way Ginkgold
- [ ] Yerba Prima Nutrimental

Yeast Infections, Women's (*See Female Problems*)

Index